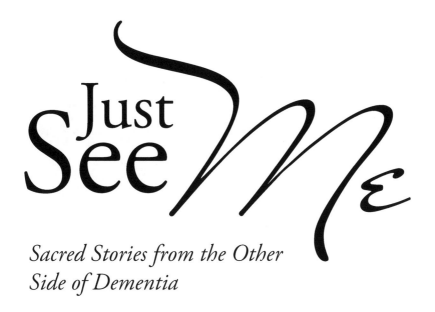

Just See Me

Sacred Stories from the Other Side of Dementia

Carmen Buck, MSN, FNP-BC

BALBOA.
PRESS
A DIVISION OF HAY HOUSE

Balboa Press books may be ordered through booksellers or by contacting:

Balboa Press
A Division of Hay House
1663 Liberty Drive
Bloomington, IN 47403
www.balboapress.com
1 (877) 407-4847

Print information available on the last page.

ISBN: 978-1-9822-0121-0 (sc)
ISBN: 978-1-9822-0123-4 (hc)
ISBN: 978-1-9822-0122-7 (e)

Library of Congress Control Number: 2018903842

Balboa Press rev. date: 03/29/2018

DEDICATION

This book is dedicated to my husband, Timothy Buck. Without your financial support, these beautiful stories would have gone untold. For this and so much more, I am eternally grateful. I inherited the entrepreneurial heart and soul from both my creative parents, as well as the grit to never give up. My heart overflows as I think of all they taught me without ever knowing it.

My grandson Kane is too young to have memories of this time but will now always have a piece of my heart to hold in his hands. May the stories inspire you to reach way high up and grab your own star over and over again.

Thirteen families told their stories to help the world learn some truths about dementia and caregiving. They demonstrate love and compassion in ways which make us all want to be better people. I carry your sacred stories in my heart, and I also dedicate this work to each of you.

FOREWORD

Pictures, photographs, snapshots, whatever you want to call them, all tell a story and represent particular moments captured in time. As a child, my father subscribed to *National Geographic* and I couldn't wait to see the amazing photographs from all over the world. I saw animals I had never seen or heard of in their natural habitats. I saw people living in ways I couldn't imagine. The colors were so vivid, the images so sharp. In my mind I created stories about what these animals and people were doing before and after the photograph was taken.

Each day, I check Instagram and Facebook to see what photographs *Carmen Buck* has recently posted. She has found a way to capture the most expressive, beautiful moments in such a touching way. In discussions with her, I know she takes dozens of photographs to find that "perfect one" that "one" that really relates to what was happening at that precise moment.

That's what a single photograph can do. It can transport you back to that particular time, allowing you to recall sounds, scents, feelings or whatever may come to mind by looking at that particular photograph. The best thing is, you can look at the same photograph a week, a month or a year later and recollect the same memory or discover brand new memories.

As someone "Living with Alzheimer's," I still look at photographs to recapture moments in time, but mostly to remind myself of the most recent events. Due to the malfunction of my short-term memory, the photos help me remember, or remember what I "think" took place.

In the 13 stories Carmen has written, she merged words with photos. The words are touching, emotional, informative, expressive, but the photographs, oh those beautiful poignant photographs, are what really tell the story. Through her lens and her creative eye, Carmen captured images that are now cherished by families who have already lost a loved one or who are now losing someone to the unknown, misunderstood monster called, "DEMENTIA!"

Seeing my Grandfather and my Mother die with Alzheimer's and my Father die with Vascular Dementia, I have a pretty good idea of what my end may look like. Between now and then, I choose to live my life as best I can. As an International Dementia Advocate, I speak to varied audiences both big and small, but my message is the same. "Just because you have a Dementia-Related Illness does not mean you have to stop living!" So . . . I don't.

I take photographs, when I remember, of things I want to remember. If I don't think of them while, "in the moment," I'll forget and that memory will also be forgotten. It's the sad truth of what Alzheimer's does. However, with people like Carmen Buck in the world taking photographs of families and people like me, the memories will live on, and for that, we should all be thankful.

I have no doubt you will enjoy this book. The stories are true, emotional yet filled with love. The photos, well the photos speak for themselves. I'll let you decide what the images are saying!

Brian LeBlanc

"I have Alzheimer's, BUT, it doesn't have me for I don't allow it to define who I am!"

'Just See Me-Sacred Stories from the Other Side of Dementia' was written so the world could witness the incredible power of storytelling, love and legacy even in the face of tragedy.

PREFACE

You might gently guide into it or take a hard fall on the pavement, but either way, becoming a caregiver is challenging. Your palms sweat, your shoulders painfully seize, you forget to breath deep, new fine lines show on your face, your chest hurts, stomach burns and yet you step forward even as your heels dig in deep. We love with intensity, and caring for someone we love takes grit, tenacity and infinite strength. We take one big step at a time all the while silently wondering; "why me, is this real and how will I possibly do this?" The grief can be palpable, but not as strong as the love which ascends from the very pain we want to avoid.

Families in *Just See Me-Sacred Stories from the Other Side of Dementia* opened their hearts and homes to share their stories of becoming caregivers to their loved ones with dementia. Lives were changed in the making of Just See Me. Truths were proudly announced and burdens were lifted. Strengths were uncovered as fears were unveiled. Tears flowed and laughter freely bounced about. Even as the stories were first told, healing began. While their stories are unique and dementia requires an extraordinary kind of caring, many of us are caregivers in our own ways.

Family caregivers can find themselves in unknown, frightful territory. Denial, imbalance and excuses scatter across every aspect of our lives. We feel achey and yet numb; empty and overwhelmed at the same time. We feel isolation, shame, lack of control, powerlessness, and profound sadness. Deep and relentless love also lives within us. Because the families in *Just See Me* opened their hearts and shared their intimate stories, I learned to love in a different more profound way even during the darkest hours.

The intention to write this book was a true epiphany. One afternoon as I finished a visit in the clinic, I heard, 'You need to tell these stories. The world needs to know.' Even with no formal education in writing, photography or business, I embarked on a venture in unfamiliar terrain with incredible certainty as every tool I needed showed up. Some may call this naive, however I'm certain it was and still is divine intervention. I discovered talents which had been buried long ago. I learned to stand in my light and speak for the truth in ways I would not have expected. Earth angels supported me. Telling these stories with the world is my sacred mission, and I was well taken care of. Only God knew there would be more to this special book, *Just See Me'* than I could imagine.

We need one another to stand strong on our own. Marcy, Bea, Tara, Jessica, Kelly, Josie, Grace, Jodi, Candy, Joy, and Tonya - you are my Earth Angels. Simply by being present, listening, accepting and purely affirming the significance of my work and art, you gave me the strength to take another step, and then another and then another.

Special thanks to my editors Joyce and Colleen with The Write Coach who helped this nurse practitioner become an author.

INTRODUCTION

Just See Me-Sacred Stories from the Other Side of Dementia

Love, transcendence and understanding exist even in the darkest moments when we look into the eyes of another and say, "I am listening."

Carmen Buck

The last 10 years of my 4 decade career as an RN and nurse practitioner were devoted to families who cared for their loved ones with dementia. They told me stories and shared memories hoping I too could see a glimmer of their loved one before dementia set in. They safely leaned on me for guidance, truth and hugs. While I had prescriptions to offer, my most appreciated gifts were presence, compassion and kindness. We laughed and cried, and I believed I had the best job in the world.

One afternoon in the middle of a busy clinic day, I heard these words: 'You need to tell these stories. The world needs to know.' After looking around to see if anyone else had heard, I walked to my office down the hall. Thankfully I had a few minutes to myself as the other 2 nurse practitioners who shared my space were not there. I've received 'downloads' or 'inspirations' previously, but never heard voices. To this day I cannot describe the voice other than it was a clear sound and message. With trembling hands, I took a piece of paper from the printer and began writing down a plan for stories which had to include images because in my mind no story is compete without pictures. I envisioned myself writing this book. It didn't seem to matter that I had no writing or photography experience beyond the ordinary. I said a prayer and asked for guidance which went something like this,"Dear God- I feel like I'm on a Mission from God like in the *'Blues Brothers'* only I know this is no joke. I'm going to need some divine intervention here. Please begin by helping me explain it to my husband." Even as I entertained myself with amusing notions, I knew I had experienced something holy. This is how my 'Mission from God,' *Just See Me, Sacred Stories from the Other Side of Dementia* was conceived about two years ago.

Worldwide, 47.5 million people have dementia, and there are 7.7 million new cases every year as of the time of this writing. H owever, these numbers fall short when we consider the impact on families and communities. Each person and every story matters. The person with dementia must learn to manage knowing little by little their memories will fade, and everyone around them must discover ways to cope as their lives change. How do we find hope as the person we love changes and slowly fades away? *"Just See Me"* helps to answer this question. Thirteen families opened their hearts and homes to give us a glimpse of their experiences with dementia-body, mind and spirit. They unknowingly described unmet basic spiritual needs. Their stories are of hope, connection, meaning, purpose, surrender, the power of prayer, humor, connection and intense love and loyalty which are all aspects of spirituality. They each have different histories, stories, and perspectives, and yet all walk the same path. You'll learn, find inspiration, and even be entertained by their stories in *"Just See Me-Sacred Stories from the Other Side of Dementia."*

I am often asked why I would want to photograph such a difficult time of someone's life. We can look at life in many ways. I choose to see every moment, whether joyful or heartbreaking as an experience to seek compassion, beauty, growth and love. God's love is everywhere, and it can be seen in the tiniest of ways. A story becomes a journey of profound connection when we can look into the eyes of another with loving intent. It feels good, like coming home when we connect with others. Welcome home!

JOHN AND PAUL

The Miracle of Prayer

**Prayer is not asking. It is a longing of the soul.
It is daily admission of one's weakness.
It is better in prayer to have a heart without words
than words without a heart."**

Mahatma Gandhi

As he sits in the same chairs and the same dining room of his parents' home, John is holding his divorce papers, along with the final paycheck for his job. His world has just crumbled around him. He sheds tears of loss, sadness, and worries because he has memory problems. Distraught, John cries to his mother over the fears no 39 year old should have, but she realizes this is the beginning of what's to come.

Mary is familiar with these fears. Her son Paul, 36, will have the same conversation with her the following year. The first of Mary's children to have been diagnosed with Alzheimer's disease, Debra, shared the same devastating news four years before John. Mary knows the course well after caring for her ex-husband who died about ten years earlier from the same terrifying disease. When I look over at Mary who keeps a constant visual vigil on her sons each carefully propped on the couch, she smiles and tells me, "I pray for a miracle that this will one day go away, and no one else will get this terrible disease. But for now, I just take care of these boys, and pray."

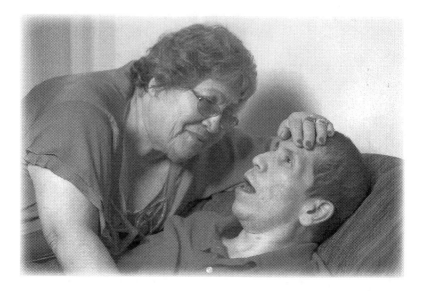

Mary and Paul

As the years went by, John and Paul became less able to care for themselves, and eventually moved into Mary's home where she, her husband and her 91-year-old mother tend to their needs. One of her granddaughters often assists on the weekends. Facility placement was an option for John and Paul, but Mary adamantly rejected it.

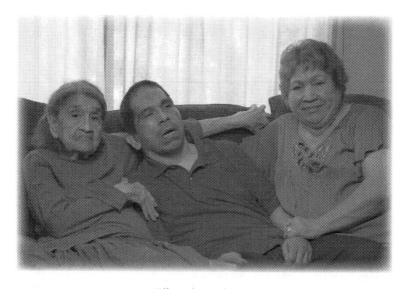

Ella, John and Mary

Debra was cared for at home before an injury resulted in long-term care placement. The decision for placement left Mary feeling powerless to manage Debra's care the way she would have if she could care for her at home. "I feel guilt about this. I used to cry all the time." She nods to her sons and says, "With Debra, I didn't have peace, but I do now because they're here with me. I pray it will stay that way, and I pray for a miracle cure. I can't give up hope because I'm their mother." Even though John and Paul cannot communicate with words, their eyes and their expressions speak volumes. Mary's face lights up when Paul smiles at her, and she returns a teasing look John gives her. She is calm, loving, and proficient in her attention. Mary was not in a state of peace when we first met, though.

> **"There is no chance, no destiny, and no fate, that can circumvent or hinder or control the firm resolve of a determined soul."**
> **Ella Wheeler Wilcox**

When I met Mary, John, and Paul in 2014 on their first visit to Seton Brain and Spine Institute in Austin Texas, our goals were to help manage the medications and the challenges of home care. The diagnoses, early onset familial Alzheimer's disease were made years prior.

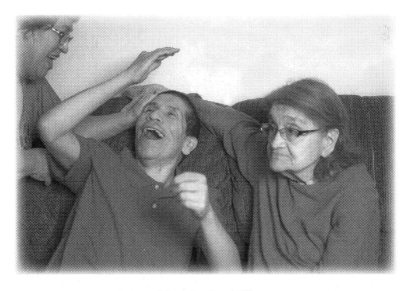

Mary, Paul and Ella

3

They came into the clinic like a storm. Paul was ever smiling and laughing. John was a bit of a flirt with his eyes and smile even though he only spoke a word or two. Paul was wheelchair bound and unable to stand on his own, and John could slowly walk down the hall with support. Mary talked so fast that I had a difficult time keeping up. This question slowed the pace of our visit and simultaneously started our journey, "What do I need to know today Mary?" It was a common question for me to ask my patients, and Mary's response was, "Oh sweetheart, you have no idea what you are asking. Listen carefully because this will go fast. I need your help, and you need to listen to me because I take care of these two boys, and nobody knows them better. I buried their father because of this disease, and my daughter is in hospice care in a nursing home now because of Alzheimer's disease. These boys," she points to Paul and John, her sons who were in their forties, "they may not be able to walk or say very much, but I know what they are trying to say to me. I know this disease. I know my boys. There is so much more you need to know. Are you ready?" I readied myself for what this fast talking, strong woman had to teach me about her life and the disease which slowly coiled around her family.

I saw them regularly over the next two years, and stood by helplessly as they continued to decline. They came into the clinic a few days after Debra died as Mary debated about whether to tell Paul and John about their sister's passing. She somehow hid her grief even while caring for her sons who needed even more of her constant attention. "One of my biggest worries is knowing some of my grandchildren could also have early-onset Alzheimer's disease." My respect for this 70-year-old grew as she became more at peace in spite of her sons' worsening conditions.

"Prayer gives me hope. I turn to God to carry my worries. I'm glad I did, too. I went through a time when I cried all the time, and I was so anxious and depressed. Do you remember when I talked so fast?" I could only nod and smile as words stuck in my throat.

Debra's death in a facility became a turning point for Mary. She fiercely resolved to care for John and Paul at home. She tells me, "I love, the kind of love a mother has; you'll do anything. I have fear too, of course, but that's when I turn to prayer. I pray all the time. I pray for a miracle and a cure, and I pray I will be able to take care of them here at home. They belong with me." Prayers give her a sense of peace and gratitude. "Doctors tell me they won't get better, but you can't take another's hope. I can still pray for a miracle even if it doesn't come for awhile." Prayer provides hope. "I can ask God for a cure, and I can ask for strength. I ask, and then I just get busy doing what I do. God lifted my worry. Prayer lifted my worry. It's in God's hands now. This is why I'm happy so much of the time. I get to love my boys.

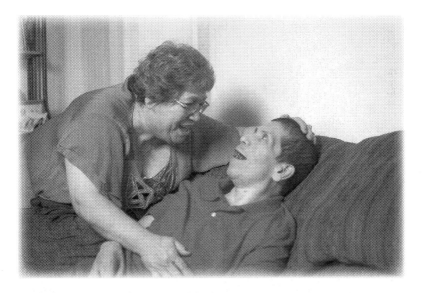

Mary and Paul

Mary is grateful she has the ability to care for her sons at home and hopes to do so until the end. They require around-the-clock care, including someone to feed them, complete help with any of the usual things needed such as toileting and bathing. I ask her what she is most grateful for, and she replied, "I can't compare what is to what it could be. I won't have 'what it could have been, so I'm grateful for now. I stay focused on that."

She stops to take a breath, and we both feel the importance of the statement she just made. It is human nature to consider what could have been, after all, it can be a recipe for sadness. Instead, Mary finds joy in the current moment. "I just love them. I take care of them, and I'll keep them at home with me as long as possible. I'm grateful I can do that. Anything else is giving up. I just can't do that."

Making an end-of-life choice for her sons has been difficult. "I don't want to give up on them, but I also need to do what is best for them," Mary tells me she signed the papers saying she doesn't want them to have cardiopulmonary resuscitation (CPR) if either John or Paul stops breathing. "That was hard, you know, but it is the right thing. They're on hospice now. That was hard too."

Mary's experience with hospice during her daughter Debra's death was not good, and she understandably avoided any talk about hospice for her sons. "It was the best thing for me. They (hospice) help so much. They are helping me to take care of them at home, and it is what I prayed for." She sheds a few tears as she describes hospice as a miracle. "I pray for miracles and hospice is one of those miracles."

Since our interview and photo session, other members of her family have been diagnosed with early onset familial Alzheimer's disease as well. Other family members have tested positive for the gene, and others have not wanted to be tested. Those under 21 years of age still have some time to decide.

Mary's family members have Familial Alzheimer's Disease (FAD), a very rare form of Alzheimer's passed down through family, inherited from a parent. This type of Alzheimer's disease accounts for between 2-3% of all cases of Alzheimer's. People with this type of dementia typically develop symptoms in their thirties or forties, which is much earlier onset than other types of Alzheimer's disease[1].

---

[1] alzheimers.net. Sauer, Alissa. "What You Need to Know About Familial Alzheimer's Disease" 19 February 2015. http://www.alzheimers.net/2-19-15-familial-alzheimers-disease/

We visit for a few minutes, and I catch a glimmer in John's eye. Perhaps he recognizes me or remembers how it felt when I used to tease and laugh with him years ago in the clinic.

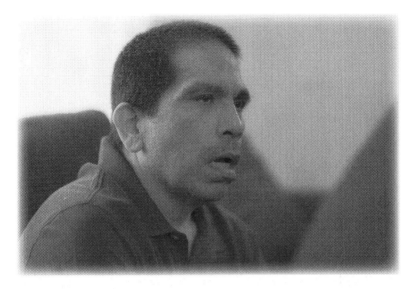

John

I watch Mary wipe around their mouths as she tells me the drooling has become worse. She talks to them as if they understand her completely. Maybe they do. She prays they do, and so do I. "This is my life. My family is my life, and my job is to take care of them and love them. Most of all, I just love them like any mother would love her children. I pray for my whole family. I learned I had to give up control over what would happen, and do my best to take care of them. I just love them. I have control over that."

AFTERWORD

Mary Paul and John

I met Mary, and her sons John and Paul in the Seton Brain and Spine Institute Neurology Clinic in Austin, TX. I lovingly referred to John and Paul as "the boys," and in the beginning, they could remember me from their previous visits. John was a quiet flirt with a sweet smile when I asked him to walk down the hall with me. It was part of my assessment, but to him, it was all ours. The look in John's big brown tearful eyes after he could no longer walk safely with me still breaks my heart.

Paul was chair bound but with an infectious laugh and ear to ear grin. The boys would laugh at one another reminding me of how they had once been. I grew to love the men who sat in front of me wishing I had known them before the disease struck.

Mary proved how faith, hope, prayer and most of all love carry her in a way only most of us dream. When I feel like slipping into the sadness or frustrations of the day, I think of Mary, and I'm magically strong again. There is a special place in my heart for Mary and her family.

DOROTHY ALBRIGHT

How We Love Her Dotisms!

"There is a thin line that separates laughter and pain, comedy and tragedy, humor and hurt."

Erma Bombeck

Laine looks around for a shaded place as she pulls her car into the parking lot. They're at a familiar local Austin park, but it is all new to her mother who sits excitedly in the passenger seat. Laine carefully unbuckles the seatbelt from around her passenger. "Mother, we're here. Why don't we walk over to the water?" she asks as she takes her mother's frail hand and guides her toward the sidewalk. Dot stops to admire the beautiful Crepe Myrtle blooms, "Oh, look at those!" She admires the flowers and foliage as it was her first visit as they maneuver to a nearby bench. "This feels so good on my legs," Dot says pointing to the spot of sunlight on her calves. Laine smiles as she thinks about the simplicity and beauty of the moment.

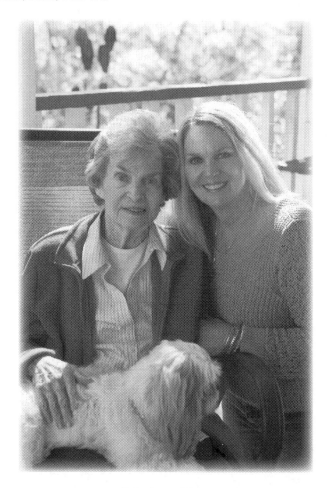

Dorothy and Laine

Her mother is too frail to go shopping; an activity enjoyed with her three daughters their whole lives. Dot was born and raised in Austin, TX but places she once loved like the University of Texas campus, the capitol building, and downtown no longer trigger the happy memories. "Austin sure has changed over the years, hasn't it?" Laine prompts. "Yes, it has. Why don't we go there?" Laine holds her mother's hand and tells her, "You are beautiful mother." After a pause, Dot looks at her and says, "I am? When I look in the mirror, I just see me." Laine smiles and is reminded to tell her sister Delinda who documents 'Dotisms,' the funny things Dot says. They silently take in the beauty of the park before Dot points once again to the crepe myrtle tree, "Look at those! I haven't seen those in a long time." They admire the beautiful purple color again as if for the first time, and Laine recognizes the blessing in her mother's shrinking world which continues to provide a constant source of joy.

> **"I always knew looking back on my tears would bring me laughter, but I never knew looking back on my laughter would make me cry."**
>
> **Cat Stevens**

Laughter escalates and seeps out the windows, under the doors and through the walls as Dot and her three daughters, Donna, Delinda, and Laine gather and retell stories of their childhood. "Mother, I ran into a friend of yours at church the other day," Delinda teases, "and you told her your Bridge game was rusty and then you won." They all giggle before Dot tells them, "Well, yes. I was good at Bridge, but I don't remember when I played last." Delinda smiles and continues," She also said you have a reputation with the group as a great Bridge player Mom." After a short pause, Dot comments, "They said that? Usually, my reputation is of me being a bad sport." Laughter erupts as they all shake their head in confirmation. "That is so true," they laugh. Dot's straightforward and honest view of her world has amplified as her dementia worsened.

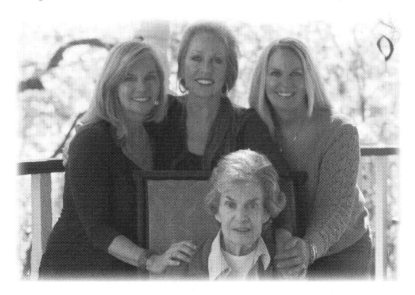

Dorothy, Delinda, Donna and Laine

The Love Story

High school sweethearts, Don and Dot met in 10th grade and were 1949 grads at Austin High. Like every epic love story, there were conflicts and challenges before they were finally able to begin their lives together. They promptly returned to Austin with Donna, their first newborn daughter as soon as Don finished his time in the military. Each of their three daughters was born five years apart.

Don was well-known for his keen sense of humor, and childlike spirit for fun. He and Dot enjoyed gatherings with friends to play cards and other games. "People just wanted to play cards with us because I had the most handsome husband." Dot teased. "And yes," Delinda finishes, "Mom told us how when she saw Daddy for the first time she said 'he was the prettiest thing she had ever seen.'" All three daughters nod in agreement as Dot laughs, "I forgot about this," and after a short pause, "well, he was." He retained his youthful sense of humor through their decades of marriage before he passed from asbestosis.

Dot stayed home to raise their three daughters, and while money wasn't plentiful, Dot was very good at managing the family budget. "I think we all learned the magic of budget by watching Mom. If we needed something or they wanted to do something, she could make it happen," Donna says. All three daughters went on to study accounting. "She made magic and not one of us could figure out how she made it work," they all laugh.

> **"Joy is what happens to us when we allow ourselves to recognize how good things really are."**
>
> **Marianne Williamson**

They all agree how Dot's temperament has changed with dementia. "We knew her personality might change with dementia, but we weren't expecting this." They laugh as Delinda explains how Dot controlled her daughters with fear, "We called it the wrath of Dot. Her words were stern." They share mutual giggles recalling a time when they were cutting up at dinner, and Dot's anger grew. "She started tapping us and warning us to stop," Delinda can barely get the words out, "We all laughed at her which was not a good idea, and then Daddy started to laugh too." The moment became a fond memory of their family united in laughter and smiles. "I wonder if Mom was as funny as we thought, or if we just laughed at her which made us all laugh more," Donna inquiries. Dot joins in the laughter before saying, "I have a lot more fun listening to them laugh about it. They have many funny stories."

The funny stories of their childhood become entwined with the entertaining statements Dot makes periodically called "Dotisms." These humorous anecdotes keep them connected and grounded as the three sisters go on with their own lives. Delinda, the youngest of the three daughters, began writing some of the statements and experiences as a way to honor their mother. Watching her mother become a more lighthearted person helped Delinda find more joy with her own family. "I'm a better mother-more attentive, caring and patient," she says. "Mother continues to teach us, even though it isn't in the way you would expect."

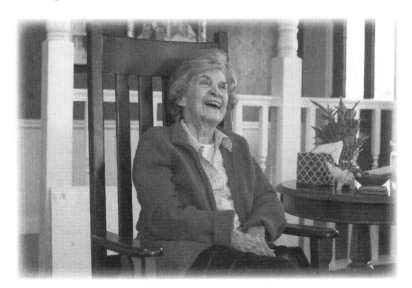

Dorothy

Donna, the eldest daughter, acknowledges the blessing of having dementia. "Life can be painful. She doesn't remember particular life pains and tragedies. Happy times and sad times come and go quickly, and the overriding feeling is how it feels right now. I recognize this and try to live more like this."

Laine, the middle daughter, isn't in full agreement. "I don't think it's a blessing." Dot forgets about their visits, accuses them of not visiting her, and experiencing angst over perceived abandonment. "She is happy and present right now, but as soon as we are gone, she won't remember our visit. We can't ever fill her need for companionship because she doesn't have her memories to fall back on. I wouldn't want to experience this because it is heartbreaking to her. Abandonment is her fear," Delaney shares. In the beginning Dot's daughters kept documentation to prove they visited, and yet she didn't believe them. She felt abandoned, and they couldn't help her. She forgets they recently visited. "We just try to focus on the here and now, and as her dementia and memory worsened, this is all she has. In some ways, it is easier. "She gets sad and lonely, but then she forgets. It's a new minute and a new day," Donna adds. "Seeing this has removed some of my fear of aging. It has comforted me." They all nod in agreement.

"All the art of living lies in a fine mingling of letting go and holding on."

Haverlock Ellis

Dot lives in an assisted living facility where she enjoys the company of others. They all experience relief and joy at seeing their mother content. They worried about how she might be as the disease progressed, and while they each love their mother, they also know they could not be her full-time caregivers. They laugh and point to one another giggling over whose home would have been best for their mother. "We all love her so much, but we all had either housing or other reasons why it wouldn't be good for her to live with us," Donna says. "It wouldn't have been easy either and we wouldn't have enjoyed her as much if we were full-time caregivers." They all nod in agreement. "She is very social and loves being with other people. She would be so bored if she lived with any of us." They all recognized their mother's needs and also how direct caregiving would've potentially ruined their relationships. "The three of us talked about this ahead of time and so glad we did," Delinda adds.

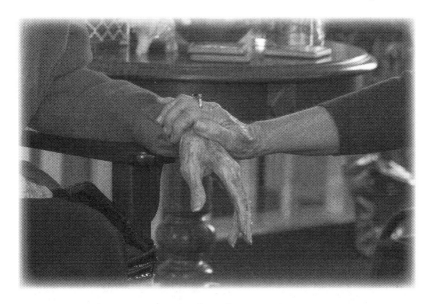

Dorothy and Donna

"Mom is fun and delights us, but she could also be a little edgy, intolerant, competitive, and inpatient. "We thought this might get worse as her condition progressed, but it hasn't worked out that way," Donna asserts. "You know what is surprising? How we're grateful she is happier now, but we all miss the less compliant, feisty mother we grew up with." They grieve the Dot who cared about her appearance and enjoyed shopping. They all smile and simultaneously look at the torn knee highs, the purse she clings to and her dress shoes as they are each remnants of the mother dementia changed.

All three daughters grieve certain aspects of their lives with Dot but are grateful for what she can offer. Donna says, "Mom doesn't have a much short-term memory, but has pearls of wisdom at the time," Donna says. Delinda nods in agreement stating, "You can bring her your issues hoping for comfort, and she is there." She smiles sheepishly, "You know it won't go anywhere because she won't remember, but she is there at the time." They laugh a little before Laine adds, "I miss talking to her and sharing. She still responds, but just not the same way as before. We are all grateful she can still empathize, but the conversation disappears when the present moment is over."

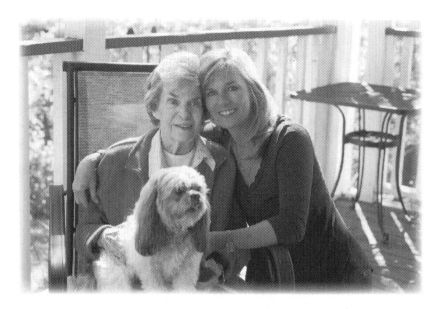

Dorothy and Delinda

We complete our time together by taking some photographs of Dot with Donna, Laine, and Delinda on the beautiful sprawling front porch. The day was chilly, but the sun shined brightly through the new leaves on the trees. I sent them the gallery so they could see the photos along with a promise to give them prints as soon as I determined which ones would be in this book. About eight months later, I had Dot's photographs and all the matting materials I needed to prepare the gifts for Dot and her daughters when my phone rang. As her daughter told me of her passing, I looked down at my hands and the smiling faces. The images, some of which later adorned her casket became priceless treasures as did the experience of joining Dot and sharing their stories. There would be no other day or time in which Dot could laugh with her daughters or pose gracefully for my camera. We all felt the simple yet extraordinary experience shared the chilly spring day with Dorothy (Dot) Albright.

AFTERWORD

$\mathcal{D}$ot, Laine, Delinda and Donna

If I had a meter to measure the love in the living room where we all gathered to talk about growing up with Dot, it would've exploded. These beautiful ladies opened their hearts to me, Dot and one another as they shared stories of the distant past and the most recent times since Dot developed Alzheimer's Disease.

They were honest, and while they didn't always share the same perspective their love and respect for their mother and each other was clear. The laughter was absolutely contagious, and we shared more tears of joy than sorrow. They talked about tough decisions and whether they were right or not. They shared their childhood memories and growing up with Dot.

I loved hearing their perspectives on how Dot's disease helped them to be better parents. Caring for their mother also led them to consider their respective futures should they also develop Alzheimer's Disease. My afternoon with these ladies was emotional, fun and nothing short of amazing.

JUANITA

$\mathcal{S}$hall We Laugh or Cry?

"Have patience with all things, but first of all with yourself."

Saint Francis de Sales

"This is my new cat," Juanita said as she greeted her daughter Dixie at the front door. "I found him in the park, and I'm teaching him to use the litter box in my room." The puppy squirmed in her arms, as she added, "He is very stubborn about it though."

Dixie was temporarily stunned into silence as she took in the situation. The urine odor in the house was a pungent indication of just how bad the litter box training was going. As the elder cat looked on, Dixie's lips slowly began to curl up toward a smile at the thought of her mother teaching a puppy to use the litter box. She simultaneously wondered how things could get this bad since her visit last month. "Mother, I think he would be happier to go outside in the yard for a little while," Dixie pressed. Juanita considered this for a moment before walking down the hall, "Well, a cat just has to learn to use the litter box. That's all there is to it." Once she retired to the bedroom with the puppy, Dixie gave in to the urge to laugh even as tears of sorrow rolled down her cheeks.

Once Juanita became engrossed in a television program, Dixie secretly ushered the puppy outside. Excusing herself, she dialed the phone, "Things are so much worse. You won't believe what happened today," she began to describe her findings and concerns to her siblings. Discussing their mother's decline was one of the many difficult conversations the five adult children have had over the past nine years. Finding a new home for the puppy was a priority, and Juanita hardly noticed his absence. Over the past nine years, Dixie and her siblings have adjusted to many changes. "The humorous moments don't happen as often, but things are going along fine now. We always expect the unexpected though," Dixie proclaims. Although Juanita has not acknowledged memory or judgment problems, she slowly allowed her five children to provide a safe and happy environment as her dementia worsened.

> **"God never gives someone a gift they are not capable of receiving."**
>
> **Pope Francis**

Dixie's Greatest Gift

Early on in the disease, a phone call from Mom's best friend was my first indication the problems were worse than I considered," Dixie explains. "Her friend and bridge partner called and told me they wouldn't play bridge with her anymore because it was too frustrating. Her memory wasn't so bad, although her decision-making was a big problem." They noticed little things, but Juanita was ingenious at covering up problems. "I was so grateful to her friend for calling me. The call was such a gift because otherwise, we wouldn't have known."

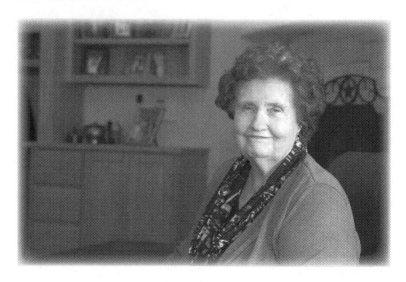

Juanita

Her dementia symptoms appeared slowly over time, taking her family by surprise. They started to notice some household and personal items missing from home. "We never found her wedding ring," Dixie recalls. "One Christmas she took the gifts from under the tree and hid them all over the place. We had to go on a hunt," Dixie adds. "At the same time, she was able to carry on in her usual way, so it was hard to know what was going on." It happened slowly, but the small frustrating things became evidence of a bigger problem. They laugh now but felt frustrated and fearful at the time.

"It's a blessing, and kind of sad too because she worried less about her belongings and stopped hiding things as her memory worsened. Mom is usually in a good mood and very sweet. Her memory is so bad she doesn't remember she was upset with us or why. We just move on to something different." Her family united to make decisions about caregivers, management of her finances, and driving. They succeeded in providing safety and autonomy while maintaining respect and love for their mother.

> **"All the art of living lies in a fine mingling of letting go and holding on."**
>
> **Havelock Ellis**

Juanita, an independent, successful businesswoman had a difficult time relinquishing her independence and lacked awareness of her shortcomings. "Giving up her car meant saying goodbye to her freedom. Taking the car away was the worst," Dixie confides. "We initially kept it, but she was not happy being a passenger while the caregivers drove. One day we removed the car completely, and it was a sad time for all of us. There is no bus system out here and after being accustomed to just getting in her car and going…" she trails off. Years have passed, and Juanita enjoys the car rides which also provide a remedy for afternoon restlessness. She no longer complains about not being able to drive herself.

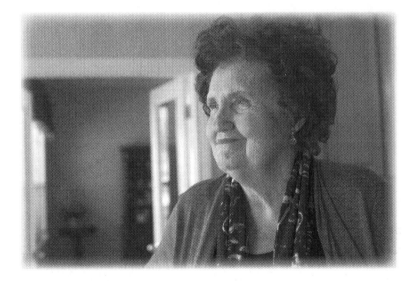

Juanita

"She enjoyed going to the movies," Dixie divulges, "but she can't follow the story line and walks out after about 30 minutes now. It's a shame because she loves movies. Instead, we watch and re-watch old television programs here at home. She doesn't know they're old or she has seen them many times before. She enjoys them every time," says Dixie. "At first we felt kind of bad about having the same programs on each day, but we've discovered the familiarity is optimal for her."

Ice cream is a favorite of Juanita's. Forgetting she has already eaten a bowl or two, she often asks her family and caregiver for more. "She has gained weight and needs new clothes often, but on the other hand, we want her to be happy. She loves ice cream, so we try to redirect and always make sure she gets enough of the healthy food too. It's just hard to know what is best," Dixie confides.

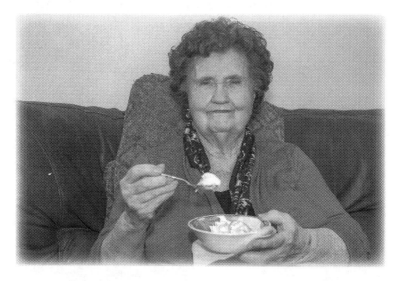

Juanita

"She took care of her father who died of dementia," Dixie continues, "We never used the word Alzheimer's because dementia didn't sound as bad to Mom. She denied having problems though, and in many ways, this made it more difficult." Although Juanita took care of her parents until they died, she has been worried about them the past few months. Believing they are still alive, she has fretted over their well being. "Dixie, I'm worried about them. I haven't heard from them since our trip to the beach. Will you call them?" Juanita asks. Her family has learned to receive her anxiety by either redirecting or being truthful. "It's surprising because she doesn't get mad when I tell her they're not here. We then just go on to something different, and she doesn't worry about it anymore. I choose my approach wisely, and if she is okay with it, so am I."

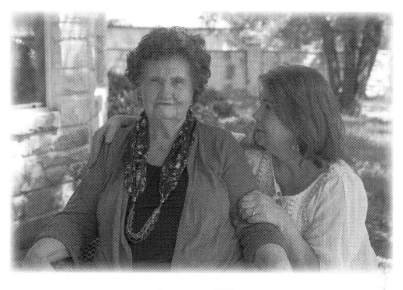

Juanita and Dixie

We Are All In This Together

Nine years passed since the revealing phone call and subsequent dementia diagnosis. Each of her five children tends to their mother's care in their own way. Juanita has around-the-clock paid caregivers in her home, and family members visit often. Knowing she wants to remain in her home, her grown children manage finances, home and yard maintenance, and caregiving needs as they arise. "We all have a role, and we let one another know if there are changes or problems. Dad taught us how we are all in this together, and we stick together even though we are all very different. There is love and respect beyond our differences," Dixie explains. Juanita joyfully recognizes all five of her grown children by name. She recognizes each of her grandchildren but is not always able to remember their names.

Don't Go It Alone

"Anyone caring for someone with dementia needs patience. They need a whole lot of it too. I'll admit I sometimes frustrated," Dixie confides. "I teach full time and visit every few weeks. Our visits are much more pleasant since I learned to visit with someone else. If I need to walk away, I can. There were times I wondered if I saw what I thought I did. Some of her comments and behaviors were strange; and I queried if I should jump in, correct or just let it go. Having someone with me helped a lot. It was okay if we both laughed."

Support groups haven't been beneficial to Dixie, but she finds comfort in conversations with other people who also care for someone with dementia. "I have a friend I talk to regularly, and although her mother is in a nursing home now, we still have so much in common. This has been most helpful for me." Dixie stresses, "It is so important to have someone to talk to [about caring for a relative with dementia]. I think it is best when they can relate to your situation."

Observing her mother's decline has been difficult for Dixie. "She is worse every time I visit, and while expected, it hurts so much to see." One of Dixie's big concerns is developing the disease. "My grandfather had dementia and now my mother. I don't know. Could I be next?" Dixie confides. "I tell my children how I don't want them to feel obligated to provide direct care. They'll need to do what is best for themselves. It's hard to be the caretaker, and I don't want it for them."

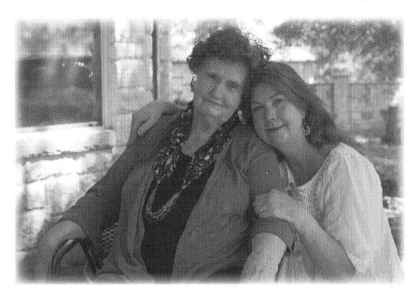

Juanita and Dixie

While Dixie and I visited, Juanita enjoyed an old western on TV and a cup of ice cream. She graciously permitted me to photograph her even though she wasn't able to remember the purpose of my visit. As our time came to a close, I thanked Juanita who was quick to offer me a scoop of vanilla ice cream. Just living isn't enough after all. One must have old westerns, a slow drive down Main Street, a Texas sunset, and vanilla ice cream.

AFTERWORD

Juanita and Dixie

I met Dixie at one of my first photography workshops. We happened to sit at the same table for lunch, and of course, the conversation of our work came up. I shared my plans to write this book, and she told me about her experiences caring for her mother, Juanita.

It didn't take long before we set a date for me to meet Juanita, talk about her experiences and treat Dixie to time in front of the camera with her mother. Photographers like Dixie spend most of their time taking pictures, so it can be a treat to be included for a change.

Her stories made me laugh so hard I cried. Her stories also hurt my heart. I loved Dixie's straightforward, unapologetic admission of preferring to visit along with someone else because her reality sometimes felt unbelievable and challenging. I drove over an hour to Juanita's home, and I was thankful because the drive home was my opportunity to cry. I cried with a sense of helplessness and with hope their story and reality would help others.

DOROTHY SOBIESKI

Moments of Grace

**"Whatever we are waiting for-peace of mind, grace,
the inner awareness of simple abundance-it will surely
come to us, but only when we are ready to receive it
with an open and grateful heart."**

Sarah Ban Breathnach

Margaret could only think of her mother. Less than twelve hours ago she received the phone call she feared. Dorothy, her mother, was critically ill and in the hospital. Quickly she left Texas and made it back to her childhood home in Michigan to see her mother one last time.

Margaret felt for the gold heart-shaped pendant, a gift from her mother, to be sure it was still there. Gently touching it was a reminder of her mother's love, and how each day with her is a gift. Margaret and her mother Dorothy lived miles apart but were very much alike. They were both strong women who believed in prayer enough to willingly release control to God. Both were lovingly blunt with opinions, took action when needed, and quick to laugh.

The stricken faces on her brother and niece greeted her. Out loud she asked, "She is dead, isn't she?" acknowledging the direct nature she inherited from her mother. "She is still with us Aunt Margaret, but is so frail," she was tearfully reassured. Margaret remained unconvinced until she could witness with her own eyes.

Margaret stopped in the doorway before taking a few tentative steps toward her mother. Dorothy's tiny, frail body lay in an intensive care bed connected with tubes and wires while the beeps and alarms associated with critical care surrounded them. Dorothy's eyes were closed as Margaret gently reached out to touch her hand, "I'm here Mama. I'm here." Dorothy cried out in pain from even the hint of caress, and Margaret's heart sank. It would not be much longer.

Going Home

Dorothy lived on her own with family support in spite of having mild dementia. Her decline had been slow, but undeniable. Her family noticed worsening memory problems, and even if she survived the hospital stay, she would not return home. Margaret prayed for her mother as well as strength to prepare for God's will.

Margaret slowly slid the key in and unlocked the door. The familiar smell of home wafted toward her providing a false sense of familiarity. Without her mother, the house was devoid of spirit and warmth, even though it looked the same as always. Margaret looked around taking stock of her mother's belongings deciding which to give away, which to discard and which to keep and wonders out loud, "where do I begin?" Even the most insignificant items seem valuable because they belonged to her mother. Taking in the energy of her mother's home, Margaret knew it would never be the same for her.

Dorothy loved her wide collection of rosaries. Each one reminded her of the important people and times in her life. As Margaret went through to set some aside for her mother, her eyes fell on a set of clear rosary beads. They captured her interest, and she tucked them away in her purse.

Dorothy miraculously survived the hospital stay and moved into a nursing home where she lived four more years. Her memory continued to deteriorate, but she usually remembered Margaret during their frequent phone calls and when Margaret was able to visit. Dorothy sometimes confused her daughter for her sister Gert. When it happened, Margaret knew not to question or correct and instead continued the conversation as Gert. While Margaret always enjoyed the visits with her mother, as time went by the moments of clarity became less frequent.

During one visit, Dorothy was confident Margaret was her sister Gert. "You've just got to go with the flow and be in their world, and if it means I am Gert for the day, then I am Gert for the day. No problem," Margaret reveals. For the day, she would be Gert for her mother. A nurse's aide entered the room and asked, "Ms. Dorothy, would you like to go to Rosary today?" Dorothy looked at Margaret and said, "Yes, sure. Would you like to go Gert?" Margaret nodded and smiled as she prepared to wheel her mother to the common room where they waited for the other residents to join them. Dorothy, as always, had a rosary with her. Margaret remembered that she had the rosary from years before still tucked in her purse. She took it out, and the short conversation to follow became one of Margaret's most fond memories of her mother.

"My that's a beautiful rosary, Margaret," Dorothy said looking at the rosary in Margaret's hands. "Maybe from a holy communion?" she continued. She paused for a moment while looking into Margaret's eyes. She then asked, "Did you take that from my house when you thought I was going to die?" She had a sparkle in her eyes, and Margaret knew her mother saw her, Margaret and not Gert. Margaret replied in the frank way they had always communicated, "Well, yes I did. Would you like it back?" She felt sheepish as if getting caught. Most importantly, however, she felt incredibly grateful for this moment of clarity with her mother and knew she witnessed a moment of grace. Her mother calmly responded, "No, you're getting use out of it. I've got this one." They sat quietly for a moment before Dorothy looked around and asked, "Gert, what's the hold up here?" Margaret had been Dorothy's daughter for one precious moment she will never forget.

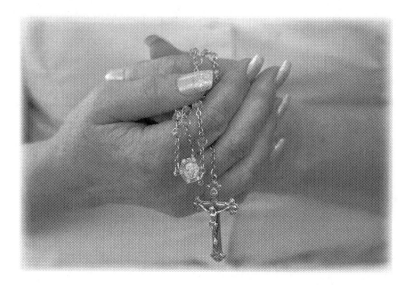

Margaret holding her mother's rosary

"Never forget the three powerful resources you always have available to you: love, prayer, and forgiveness."

H. Jackson Brown, Jr.

Dorothy had occasional moments of clarity Margaret refers to as "moments of grace" because they often occurred around times of prayer. Nursing home life is not always pleasant, especially for a woman like Dorothy who was successful, active, and social. "I don't feel useful, Margaret. I don't work or cook. I don't do anything around here because they do everything for me. My family doesn't need me anymore," Dorothy confided. Margaret held her hand and her gaze before giving her perhaps the most supreme gift of all. "Mom, you've got the greatest power over all of us. You can pray for us. You can pray all day if you want. This is the best thing you can do for us. It has always worked," Margaret said looking into her mother's eyes unaware of the gift she had just given. A life devoid of purpose and meaning can be lonely and sad. Dorothy smiled knowing her family needed her after all. She was still able to take care of her family. Margaret smiled with tears in her eyes, as she shared this story with me, "Her memory was so poor, but she remembered it was her job to pray for all of us, and it changed everything for her."

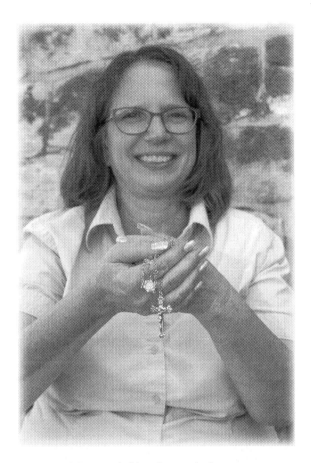

Margaret holding her mother's rosary

Her family honored Dorothy at her burial by sharing memories she had lost along the way. They found themselves laughing with joy and lost in the stories memorializing the woman they loved so. Rather than the tradition of throwing dirt onto the casket, they threw Double Mint gum packages because Dorothy loved her double mint gum. Margaret held her rosary tight thanking God for the special moments of grace she had with her mother and for the family who surrounded her with love and laughter.

AFTERWORD

Margaret and Dorothy

I met Margaret at a women's business networking meeting as I cruised around still very uncomfortable at meetings where I know no one. At the time, I had a hard time describing what I do. I'm a photographer, writing a book about families with dementia because I like helping people create their legacies and I've been a nurse for almost forty years. It can be very complicated, and any new entrepreneur can relate.

Margaret, with her warm, welcoming smile showed me her 'Thirty-One' bags, and we struck up a conversation. Just a smile and a few friendly words and I no longer felt alone. When she heard about my business and mission, she asked if she could tell me about her mother, the rosary, a moment of clarity. The significance of those few moments had me hooked. I hadn't decided if I would include any stories if the loved one with dementia had passed, but Margaret made the decision easy.

GRACETTA FORBES

A Visionary for Compassionate Action

"God wants us to know that life is a series of beginnings, not endings. Just as graduations are not terminations, but commencements. Creation is an ongoing process, and when we create a perfect world where love and compassion are shared by all, suffering will cease."

Bernie Siegel

Gracetta stepped out onto the porch and examined her white glove-laden hands. She enjoyed visiting her daughter's homes and walking about the neighborhoods. She held her head up high, smiled at the clouds and brushed away the worries about finding her way home. A prayer passed her lips as she took the steps off the porch and began her walk. Later that evening as the sugar dissolved into her tea, she shared the weight of her worry with her daughter before suggesting, "The house across the street is for sale. It is one story, and I think we should buy it. I believe it is time for me to get one of those medic alert bracelets, too." The first of many difficult conversations.

Vashti Jude and Vidette, Gracetta's daughters, began to notice their mother's memory problems about a decade ago, but nobody wanted to make it real by saying it out loud. "Not my mother. She was the glue holding us all together. She was always my lifeline," Vidette confided. "I couldn't't allow myself even to imagine what would happen. Not one of us could manage without her because she took care of all of us. This just could not happen." Gracetta cared for her husband who suffered from a variety of military-related ailments while attending support groups for people with mild cognitive problems. She continued her favorite activities and refused to let dementia define her. Vidette smiles, "Momma was so curious and wanted to know more. People thought she was the caregiver and not the one with memory problems." Vashti Jude and Vidette exchange a conspiratory look as they confided in the revelation. Their mother could not be present for them as she always had, and they would need to find their way. More than a decade has passed since these very dark days.

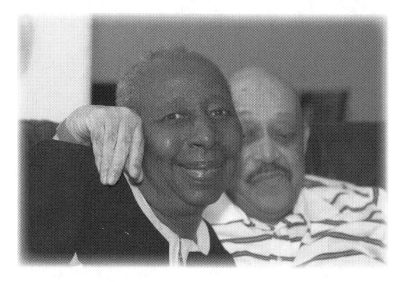

Gracetta and her husband Booker

"Too often when embarking on a journey, we focus on what needs to get done without looking at who we need to become in order to get there."

Cheryl Richardson

Gracetta, the youngest of ten children, was born Grace Etta in southern Louisiana. She changed her name because she felt Gracetta was more befitting her style and personality. Gracetta knew she was one of a kind and spent a good bit of her life encouraging other women to stand in their own light as she had.

"Momma inspired so many people to be successful for themselves, but they also wanted to please her," Vidette tells me proudly. Her daughters fondly recall Gracetta's solo road trips even during times of civil unrest in the south. She recognized her right to enjoy the freedom of the wind in her hair and sights of a new place at a time when many women didn't drive at all. Fellow military wives gathered around her to learn how to manage their money, drive, and take care of themselves. This sharp, proper, intelligent, financially savvy eloquent speaker was clearly ahead of her time. She was also the queen bee to her family and even her older siblings. Gracetta led with compassionate action guided by her curiosity, creativity, and love. She was the core of life and very root to her husband and daughters' successes while quietly earning the respect of those around her.

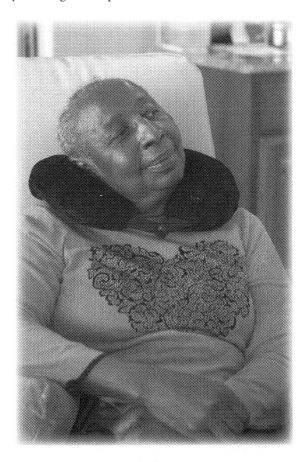

Gracetta

> **"Love begins at home, and it is now how much we do, but how much love we put in that action."**

Mother Teresa

Witnessing Gracetta's slow cognitive fade made her daughters even more adamant to create a loving environment for her. "Coping skills you thought you had are not enough because making difficult decisions amplifies every conflict-even those saved up for 50 to 60 years. There is no escape and the one person I needed most couldn't help me," Vidette explains. Vashti Jude and her sister were united in the desire to care for their mother, but not always in the execution of the plan. Both women are advance practice nurses with strong, confident personalities who discovered the pain of solving difficult problems in the midst of a crisis. With laser sharp desire to care for their mother, they found solutions and managed to heal their wounds.

Vashti Jude and Vidette's Success Solutions

The formula Vashti Jude and Vidette developed to care for their mother was born through a painful process with many ups and downs. They yearned to respect their father's desire to care for Gracetta at home but quickly recognized this was not the best for their mother. He also needed help, and the girls were forced to investigate care for both of their parents who each had different needs. They hungered to provide an inner and outer environment suited for her while giving her decision-making control for as long as possible.

Over the last ten years, Gracetta has become less able to express her wishes, but they are sensitive to her needs by making sure things are in alignment with her wishes. They and the three full-time caregivers who care for Gracetta tune into her needs, body language, and moods. "They probably don't like me, but they tolerate me. Momma comes first, and I'll do or say whatever it takes for her to be happy. Things have to be perfect, or they hear from me," Vidette declares.

Gracetta's carefully chosen caregivers maintain a consistent schedule. They repeatedly demonstrate their love as they take Gracetta on errands that end with a stop for her favorite treat. They recognize her facial expressions and quickly attend to her needs with respect, kindness, and the reverence she deserves. I couldn't help but notice the joy in Gracetta's smiles when her caregiver Sara offered her affection. Vidette and Vashti Jude concede they are blessed to be able to provide this for their mother and give credit to their mother's skillful money management through the years. Vashti Jude admits, "She didn't know she was saving for her long-term care, but because she did, we can provide this home and caregivers."

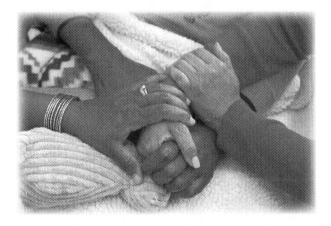

Forbes Family

Clutter can result in confusion for people with dementia and the caregivers maintain a clutter-free home for Gracetta. She lives in the downstairs of a large two-story home, while her caregivers stay in the upstairs rooms. The area is open with plenty of natural light and views of the backyard. The floor is uniformly colored because darker colors can make it look like there is an opening in the floor. The caregivers and her daughters walk with her slowly and carefully inside and outside of the home.

A tangible sense of peacefulness permeates the home. Gracetta enjoys music, and her favorite sounds fill the silence. Gracetta's sense of humor, laughter, and playfulness are honored by all who enter. Conflict is part of life, but they are careful to avoid tension in her presence.

Vashti Jude and Vidette came together to care for their mother and ailing father through acceptance, negotiation, and reconciliation. After years of trial and error, they created a world with love, support, security, and control. They remembered the values their mother instilled in them, put family first and never gave up on one another. They solved problems with love and the compassionate action their mother so often demonstrated.

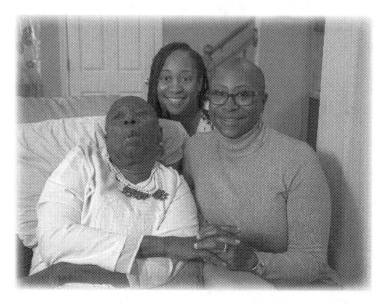

Gracetta, Vidette, Vashti Jude

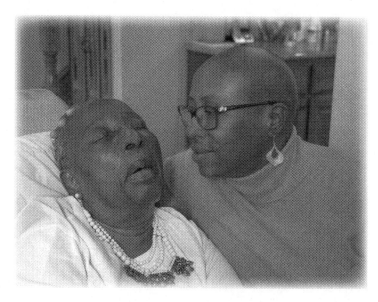

Gracetta and Vashti Jude

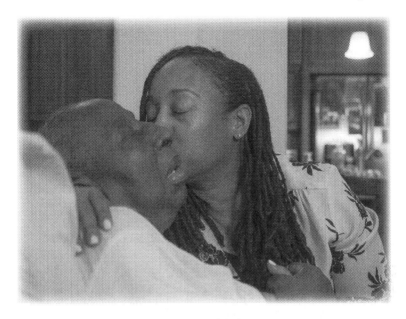

Gracetta and Vidette

I recently visited with Vashti Jude and Gracetta to deliver their portraits. She looked much the same as she did a year ago. She smiled as Vashti showed her the portraits, and this instant of recognition continues to be a source of joy for her family and for me. We were fortunate to catch it on video. Dementia is a progressively debilitating disease, and Gracetta's fortitude is certainly a testament to the power of family, love, thoughtful caring, and her beautiful spirit.

AFTERWORD

Gracetta, Vashti Jude and Vidette

"Coincidence is God's Way of Remaining Anonymous."

Albert Einstein

There's nothing quite like a piping hot pizza in the midwinter sunshine of Central Texas. Marcy, a physician's assistant, and I hardly noticed guests on the patio because we were deep in conversation about the end of my long nursing career and the beginning of this book. We debated the virtues of pursuing a dream versus a job with security. As we discarded our empty pizza trays, a woman sitting near us called to us, "I don't mean to eavesdrop, but I heard you talk about long hours and hospitals. You must be nurses. I recognize the lingo. I'm Vashti Jude and I'm a nurse too. So is my sister." We introduced ourselves and the conversation veered in the direction of my plan to write a book sharing stories of family caregivers to those with dementia. Vashti's eyes teared up. "My mother has dementia, and she lives real close to here. I would love to learn more about your project." It wasn't long before I set a date to visit with Gracetta, her daughters and caregivers.

I visited and photographed Vashti Jude, Vidette, Gracetta and her caregiver Sara, and returned another day to photograph Gracetta and her husband. I delivered their photos months later, and the look of awareness and joy on Gracetta's face became forever printed in my memory and my heart. I had only my cell phone with me, but was able to get a few video clips. It's

40

one of my favorites though. These goose bumps or 'God-bumps' moments happen to remind me that life is so much bigger than I could ever imagine. You can view 'Gracetta Recognizes Love' here: http://bit.ly/Gracetta

On March 8, 2018, after sharing her love and life with her family and others for 77 years, while in the loving arms of her daughters, Gracetta peacefully passed. They sang the gospel music she loved, prayed, and laughed while reminiscing cherished family memories. I attended her memorial with a full heart knowing she lived and died surrounded by love.

JUDE W.

The Bigger the Love, The Bigger the Hurt. But, the Bigger the Love

"Each relationship has at its heart a holy purpose."

Doreen Virtue

At 78 years old, Jude and his wife Beth, 63 always loved sitting outside and watching the clouds. With comfort in the silence, they sit, hold hands and look at the sky. One afternoon, Jude broke the silence, "I think I would love to get married," he smiled at her. She returned his smile, and said, "Oh, Jude. We are already married. See, here is my ring," she paused and pointed, "and here is your ring." She sweetly reminded him they were married 23 years ago. He nodded at her before resuming his careful examination of the clouds. Later in the evening, Beth thought about the conversation and decided to bring their wedding album to show him about their life together. Finding ways to trigger his memory in spite of worsening dementia was important to Beth.

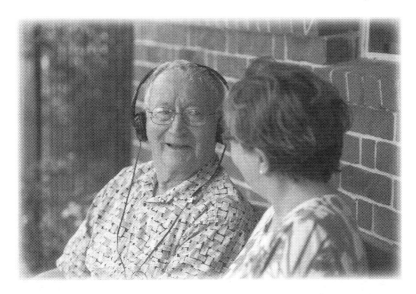

Jude and Beth

The next day she proudly showed Jude their album, prompting his memory of the big day. Staring blankly at the people in the photos, he pointed to a photo of himself, and asked, "Who is this?" Dementia took his ability to recognize himself, and Beth realized she had made a mistake. Looking at the photos only deepened the wound created by the many losses. Later in the evening, as she helped the facility staff wash the dinner dishes, she made a pact with herself to gracefully and joyfully accept his proposal should he ask again. The next time he asked her, she agreed to marry him, and his smug and endearing response was all she needed to know the future would carry wounds as well as moments of grace and healing.

Her eyes filled with tears as she shared this story. We sat in silence for a few beats before she said, "He doesn't ask me anymore, though. He isn't able to talk well. This is when I wish I didn't feel so much. The bigger the love, the bigger the hurt. But, the bigger the love. Look at what I've got, though. I may have a big hurt, but it's okay because I have this big love."

**We need to find God, and he cannot be found in noise
and restlessness. God is the friend of silence. See how
nature - trees, flowers, grass- grows in silence; see
the stars, the moon and the sun, how they move in
silence... We need silence to be able to touch souls."**

Mother Teresa

Beth and I sat in silent reverence as Jude silently walked among the other
residents at The Cottages of Chandler Creek, a memory care facility. He
was generous with his smile and occasionally walked up to other residents
in the memory care facility, silently stood before them as if asking for
permission before placing his hands on their head or shoulder in soundless
prayer. He would occasionally quietly whisper, "bless you, my child." He
gravitated toward those who seemed to need the comfort the most. Jude
is a former Roman Catholic Priest who left the priesthood at age 50. This
was when Jude's life became rich in ways he couldn't imagine.

At the age of 14, Jude left his family home to join the seminary. He was
born and raised in a small, poor farming community where the parish
priest was his only role model other than farming. Choosing the priesthood
for this kind, gentle man was not a mistake, although there came a time
for him when he yearned for a different kind of life. After receiving his
master's degree in counseling, he grew a private practice. For 15 years he
was also the director of a retreat house where he loved the informal setting.
His many clients adored him and how he touched their lives.

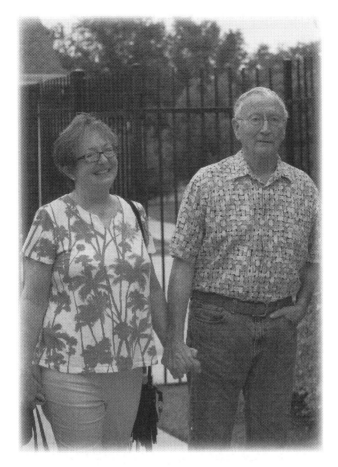

Jude and Beth

We Are Partners For The Whole of Life

"When you dance, your purpose is not to get to a certain place on the floor. It's to enjoy each step along the way."

Wayne Dyer

Along the way, he and Beth's friendship flourished to a profound and respectful love. She was finishing her master's degree while Jude adjusted to life outside the priesthood. He had to learn to support and take care of himself in ways the priesthood did not prepare him. He had never owned a car, paid for insurance, ironed a shirt or lived independently. After five years, their relationship became romantic. He looked forward to being a stepfather and was known to say he inherited love when they married. They faced a variety of sacrifices resulting in a strong marriage filled with love, appreciation, and respect for one another beyond measure.

Beth first perceived changes in Jude's behavior around 2006. There were some mild memory problems, but changes in his judgments were most disconcerting. The decision to abruptly close his thriving counseling practice in 2006 was a surprise to Beth. Other types of work helped him stay busy, but the lapses in judgment and insight became painfully clear to Beth, their friends, and colleagues. Jude seemed unaware of his deficits, resulting in Beth second guessing herself. Perhaps the unusual behaviors were secondary to his alcohol consumption which had become a problem at times or was he using the alcohol to self-medicate? In spite of being familiar with the signs and symptoms of dementia, alcohol consumption made it difficult for her to know what was happening. Years later Jude was diagnosed with mild cognitive impairment, which can be a pre-curser to dementia. It is likely high intelligence and familiarity with the tests contributed to a delay in diagnosis but continued decline led to an eventual diagnosis of dementia.

> **"How did find some peace with the decision about memory care for Jude? I realized I couldn't be the wife he needs if I'm his caregiver too. It took some time for me to accept this. Our relationship comes first."**

> **Beth**

Beth cared for Jude at home until it became too difficult to manage alone. Choosing a memory care facility to partner with her in Jude's care was a priority and a challenge. Learning to navigate the role changes between wife and caregiver as Jude's condition worsened resulted in the awareness of being wife and caregiver for all things was unhealthy for her. Beth, as a social worker and professional caregiver, believed loving someone means caring for them when needed. Devotion to Jude as his condition worsened meant considering the unthinkable. A conscious decision to separate being his wife from the role of caregiver led her to make the heartbreaking decision to release some of Jude's care to the facility staff. "I can be the wife and they can't. So, I'll be the wife." Some bathing, grooming, and dressing tasks were slowly turned over to the team while Beth enjoys time being Jude's loving partner. The decision to choose an early retirement from work was apparent. "He deserves more than my leftover time. Jude does not get my leftover time."

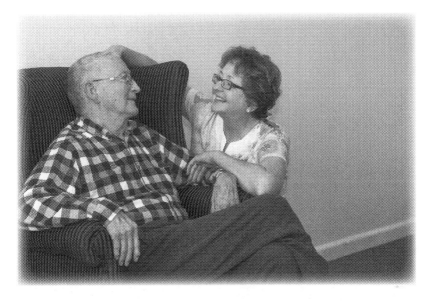

Jude and Beth

"The ultimate measure of a man is not where he stands in moments of comfort and convenience, but where he stands at times of challenge and controversy."

Martin Luther King, Jr.

The Hardest Part

Jude knows Beth is important to him. "He recognizes I'm a good thing. He might know me as Beth but probably not as his wife." Knowing he is her Jude has helped to accept life as it is. "The most painful thing is when he tries to tell me something, and I just can't decipher it. If I'm not sure what he says, my responses are noncommittal like 'that's interesting.' But when he wants to tell me something, and I just can't get it, he grows silent. Those times I just cuddle and hold him." Finding uninterrupted private time to cuddle is a challenge of facility life. The request to knock before entering is often, but not always respected. Beth sighs, "I really miss being alone with him."

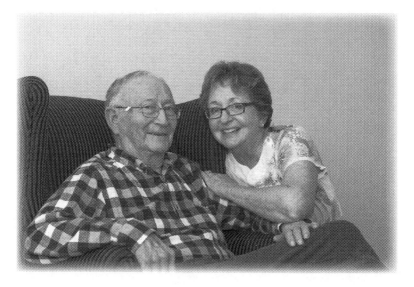

Jude and Beth

Beth's Bag of Tricks

Something sweet is the first of the contents of Beth's bag to show itself. "Jude likes snacks." An iPod with a playlist of his favorite songs and a headset is close behind. To create this playlist, Beth went through his old albums from a time before they met. "When I made this, he wasn't able to tell me which songs he liked best, so I had to figure it out. The music gives us something to enjoy together." Wooden building blocks are the next of the bag items. Jude loves to tinker, and while he cannot put things together, he can take them apart. "He focuses on taking it apart, while I make a whole new one for him. We can do this for hours." They spent their days enjoying simplicity as always love. Defining their love only through the eyes of dementia would be a mistake. Their relationship has been and remains multifaceted even as they cope with managing the disease. Beth looks forward to one day reflecting on this time of their lives and seeing the value in the challenges. The disease has brought pain, but Beth wishes to focus on the resulting growth and happiness.

> **"Patience is not simply the ability to wait - it's how we behave while we're waiting."**
>
> **Joyce Myer**

On visits, Beth immerses herself into his world. She realized the only way to enjoy their time together was to be in his world. When visitors come and see him, the best thing they can give him is attention and to go with the flow. "We can't forget people with dementia are people. Nobody is perfect, and we learn along the way how to love and care for one another as things change. In this case, we need to walk alongside them in their world and not make them fit into ours."

Beth looked out the window and said, "I have one last thing to share." She smiles and wipes away her tears. "In the beginning, it was so hard for me to leave him at night, and he insisted on going to the window and kissing me through the window. He stayed at the window waving goodbye and kept waving as I drove away. It seemed like a horrible thing to do to me. I dreaded it because it was already hard to leave him." She pauses and looks out the window again before saying, "I dreaded it then, but now I wish he could do it again. I don't have it now, and I want it, even just one more time."

AFTERWORD

Jude & Beth

Jude was a resident of the Cottages and Chandler Creek, a memory care facility, and their executive director MaryJane Kesler referred Beth to me. I'm so grateful she did! It can be uncomfortable to meet someone and quickly begin an in-depth conversation about their experiences living with dementia, their marriage, and life-changing decisions but Beth and I effortlessly connected. I believed we recognized the compassion in one another.

Beth was open, warm and drew from her career as a social worker. A few hours into our conversation, she looked at me and said, "You know, I can't even remember everything we talked about." A day or two later she emailed me asking me to be sure and focus on their love and their relationship and how dementia did not define their love. She couldn't have realized how clear this was to me early in our talk.

I was there when Jude moved into a different memory care facility, Poet's Walk in Round Rock, and witnessed Beth's agony over difficult decisions. I've been blessed to photograph this beautiful couple exchange loving looks even as Jude's condition declines. Dementia does not define the love Beth and Jude share.

DAVID R.

The Poverty of Isolation

"Isolation is the sum total of wretchedness to a man."

Thomas Carlyle

"Is he coming over today?" David asks Joan pointing toward a picture of his best friend. She chooses her words carefully knowing the answer will hurt him, and in ways, he won't be able to express. "No David," she pauses, "I know this is hard for you, but he isn't." She kindly tells him how people don't visit or call anyone. Joan hopes his diminishing memory will protect him from repeated heartbreak. "My friends were taken away," he tells her. She nods to him while giving me a conspiratorial glance. "It's a cruel thing," she confides. "I get so angry about how people have abandoned us. I don't understand your book title about love living here because there is no love here. This disease has left us alone in our world."

David still remembers how he felt 15 years ago when he started to notice. Always a lover of words, he enjoyed thoughtful discussions about interesting topics. "I didn't know what to expect," he described the problems he had writing and processing words. Words brought him delight in writing, reading, and learning. "I was so afraid when I couldn't write," he stuttered after a long pause, "I thought it was the end, but it kept happening." Much of David's speech is halted making conversation difficult to understand.

As a successful journalist, David effortlessly chronicled events. He grieves the ease in which he could once write and express his thoughts and feelings. He mourns the loss of strong bonds and connections he built with others through the years. David's ability to communicate deteriorated along with the relationships he once cherished. Joan isn't sure why people avoided them at a time when she and David needed them so much. "Was it because he needed more help or was challenging to understand? What kinds of people run away when you need them most? It has been terrible."

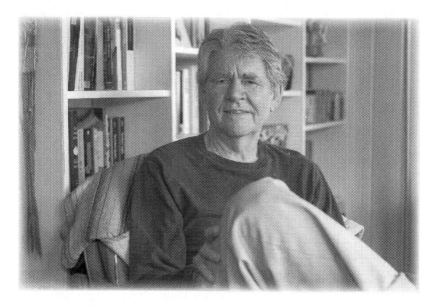

David

"We may encounter many defeats, but we must not be defeated."

Maya Angelou

Countering his pain, David enjoys attending the local AGE program (Austin Groups for the Elderly) four days a week. Joan, aging herself, is still able to drive him there. He relishes in entertaining others with his harmonica playing and enjoys many of the activities. Joan confesses, "He enjoys it. You know what's painful- watching my intelligent, articulate husband struggle with simple group activities. I'm glad he likes it because I need the break. I drop him off and leave. It's all so very hard." She perks up before offering. "One other attendee only spoke Japanese and couldn't join in with the others. He just stood up, walked over to her and began counting in Japanese. I was surprised! We took a semester of Japanese in college, and I don't remember a word, but David just started counting with her. It was incredible. Maybe he recognized some of his loneliness in her. It was beautiful," she pauses. "In fact, we have encountered more support and kindness from others with dementia than we did from our friends."

Reading is one of David and Joan's favorite pastimes. While it is a challenge for him to follow the written word, he still enjoys recorded books. Sadly, as time goes by, he has more difficulty following the stories. "There are many losses. Reading, writing, and pretty soon even listening to stories will be out of reach. She shakes her head, "I'm not sure he even realizes it now. I will though," Joan shares knowing David's love of books is another mutual joy released from their lives.

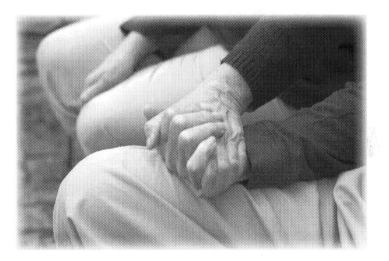

David and Joan

David loves to play his harmonica, and it has become one of his best means of communication. Their dog Luna listens attentively at his side as he plays his tunes. Converse to his speech, his music is melodic, free and fluid. Joan enjoys the music, but the real joy comes from his loving smile at her and the light in his eyes. Consumed with delight and fear Joan watches her husband communicate in the best way he can.

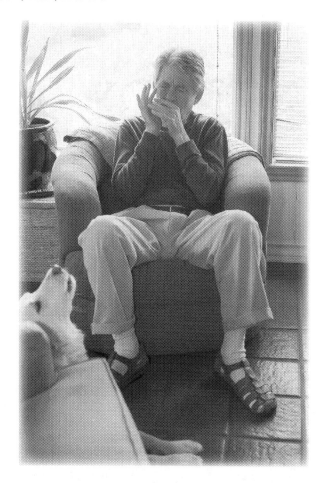

David and Luna

"It's difficult to admit to ourselves that we suffer. We feel humiliated like we should have been able to control our pain. If someone else is suffering, we like to tuck them away, out of sight. It's a cruel, cruel conditioning. There is no controlling the unfolding of life."

Sharon Salzberg

Married fifty-one years, Joan's ability to sense and experience her husband's anguish is understandable. She carries a heavy load of worries. As one might expect, Joan noticed David's problems long before he mentioned anything to her. "He drank back then. He drank more and more as time marched on and things became worse. I didn't know what came first. Did he drink because he couldn't handle the problems or was the alcohol the cause? It was very frustrating. There was such a mix of emotions and fear."

As time went on, Joan became responsible for all household maintenance and finances. "This house feels huge. There is a lot to do, and it is too much sometimes. I've had health problems, and I'm not sure how long I'm going to be able to take care of him." she tells me as we all stroll about their beautifully flowered yard. David points to a gate and after giving him a pause Joan fills in, "he built this for us. He enjoys the peace outside." His smile is as bright as the sun, and he is happy to stop for a quick picture or two.

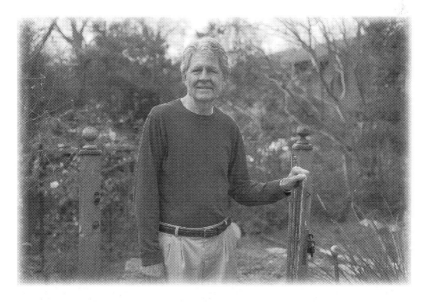

David

Joan and David, once avid travelers, are no longer able to visit their son who lives in Scotland. "Our son Kristan, and his family are lifesavers. They are all the way in Scotland, but every Sunday dinner, they sit the computer at the table, and we share a meal," Joan relates the best remedy for the pain of dementia and isolation. They share updates and relish in their grandchildren's stories. Regular calls and emails to her son and daughter-in-law are valuable. "It has to be difficult for them to be so far away from us," Joan says.

Attending AGE and their regular family calls helped Joan and David with their feelings of isolation, but the agony over losing lifelong friends and some family members is palpable. "I don't even know why they stopped coming by or calling. We're still here. David knows they don't call or visit. It hurts and yet they're too afraid or whatever it is. I don't know, but it feels awful for us. I can't be everything for him." She waits for a beat before saying words she no doubt hoped she would never need to declare, "I have some big decisions to make, and I'm looking into placement at a veteran's home. It's just too much for me." Joan and her son are left to make the painful decision about moving David into a home not their own. After decades together, they would be apart. Joan contemplates with anger and fear about what is best for David as well as her well being. David quietly pets Luna's head not revealing how much he understands. As our visit drew to a close, I wondered if sharing her story would bring Joan peace or more angst.

> **"Could a greater miracle take place than for us to look through each other's eyes for an instant?"**
>
> **Henry David Thoreau**

One Year Later

After completing all the interviews and photo sessions for this book, it was time to deliver David and Joan's portraits. I looked forward to catching up and meeting Kristan who was in Austin visiting. A jubilant Joan answered the door, smiling and offering hugs. Luna once again welcomed me to a home apparently missing David's presence.

Kristan is in Austin to visit with his parents and helping his mother transition his father to a nursing home. Caring for David at home was no longer a good option for Joan who has health problems. This visit with his parents would be both joyful and distressing.

Having heard about their Sunday Skype dinners, I was eager to learn Kristan's experience as an adult child living far away from aging parents and a father with dementia.

"I felt such guilt and powerlessness. I didn't know how to help them. We saw the decline remotely. It was even harder for my mother I'm sure. I knew she couldn't handle it, and I wanted to take care of both of them. It was impossible," he declares.

Joan reassures, "Just being able to talk to you whenever I needed was such a relief." Kristan remained relatively unconvinced, "Well, it wasn't enough, but it was all I had. The Skype calls helped to create a little normalcy to the family environment for Mom and Dad and us. It's a surrogate for the experience but not as good. The kids could see changes in Dad, and it was tough for me as both the father and the son. I could see them snicker if Dad forgot something. I told them to stop, and on the other hand, I knew if I were their age I would snicker too. He said something funny, and who knows how to act? Then I would get upset at my reaction. There was no winning," he confided as Joan conceded the significance of the weekly video calls. "It was hard to have that normalcy, but we did our best."

Joan recalls our first visit and the anger she felt over being a caregiver for her husband with dementia. "Caring for him was difficult, and then when his friends and family stopped visiting, it was horrific," she began. "I'm sorry if I wasn't very nice. I just couldn't understand how you could tell me there is any love with this terrible disease. I think I see now, but," she smiles, I'm still not sure how our story can help others." Knowing the pain isolation brings many caregivers, I gently reassured her, "when we recognize ourselves in someone else's story, we no longer feel quite as alone Joan."

The very story that brought such sorrow to Joan a year ago was plainly a part of her healing journey, and I joyfully retired the concerns of our first visit as we hugged goodbye.

AFTERWORD

David and Joan

David was a patient of mine, and I had seen him a few times at Seton Brain and Spine-Neurology Clinic. David had been a writer and enjoyed the arts, and suffered with speech problems. When I arrived at their home, he, with Joan's prompts was happy to introduce me to their dog Luna, play his harmonica and listen as Joan and I talked. He did his best to contribute although he had a difficult time pronouncing and putting words together.

Joan was angry. She was lonely and feeling isolated from friends and family. She made it clear how the word "Love" didn't belong in a title of a book about dementia. The book's original title was *Love Still Lives Here*. Living with dementia and the multiple challenges of living with dementia was a strain on their lives, their dreams, and their marriage. She repeatedly told me, "I can't imagine how our story could help anyone else." She didn't realize her pain and frustration with isolation is shared by so many.

Our second visit a year later gave me the opportunity to meet their son Tristan and embrace Joan who was feeling much more at peace. I am grateful for Joan's honesty when describing the raw pain of isolation. We know she is not alone, and her journey gives us hope.

FAY LASITER

"Daddy, It's Me. I Will Always be Here."

"Fear is a natural reaction to growing closer to the truth."

Pema Chodron

Vicki is grateful to be driving away from the congested Austin city traffic. After working all night, her mind buzzes with worry about her father, Fay Lasiter, who always goes by 'Lasiter.' She is exhausted. He has been confused, paranoid, and determined to keep loaded guns with him at all times. Bizarre behaviors have become more common and extreme. The daily scene is never quite the same at her father's home.

"Uncontrolled chaos," she thinks out loud, "My life is uncontrolled chaos." Uncontrolled chaos in her mind and life is about to propel her into a time of profound fear and pain. If Vicki knew who to pray to, she would pray for the chaos to end and to have her loving father back with her. Instead, she takes a deep breath of courage and opens the door to her father's home.

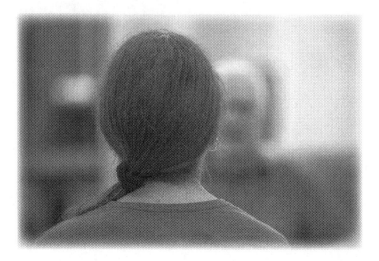

Fay and Vicki

"Daddy it's me," she calls. "Daddy it's Vicki, and I'm coming in" she repeats slowly and clearly as she opens the front door. Lasiter is standing in the middle of the living room holding a gun in his underwear. Her 89-year-old father is lost in his home again. Drawers are open and contents spilled out. As he calms down, gently she removes the loaded firearm while guiding him to his bedroom to find some clothes. The coffee cup is on the stove, and she makes a mental note to remove it soon noting his new habit of heating coffee on the stove.

As Vicki and Lasiter share breakfast, she looks into the eyes of the man who has always been there for her. How he maintains a full head of beautiful hair and his sharp wit even at nearly 90 continues to amaze her. Through the years he worked hard and never felt enough because of his limited education. However, she sees an incredibly intelligent man who far surpasses his third-grade education and took good care of his family.

Holding the wrinkled and gnarled hands, the same hands which dutifully and lovingly cared for her mother for two years before her death, Vicki returns the smile. They always have each others' backs no matter what. Now it is her turn to have his. She rises from the table and opens the blinds to let the light shine into the disheveled home. The reality is her loving father has become paranoid and easily angered in a home he is no longer able to keep repaired and cleaned. She wants to take him to the doctor, but he resists. Often, she wonders what to do next, while grieving every little loss along the way.

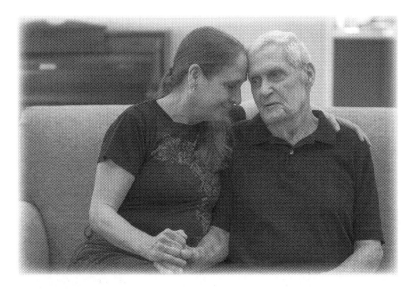

Faye and Vicki

Vicki does not resist the truth something is wrong, but she has no idea what to do other than deal with the day to day. "Daddy," she says, "do you want to talk about the guns?" He reaches for her hand and says, "I'm sorry Vicky. I don't know what gets into me sometimes. You tell me it's not real, and I believe you, but it seems real. It seems real." She'll wait another day to decide what, if anything, to do. The tears welling up in her eyes will be allowed to fall later when she gets home. She smiles at this man she loves so much as she prepares to go home and sleep a few hours before doing it all again. She feels immense gratitude she still has her Daddy to hug.

Year One: Madness

Year Two: Madness, the Sequel

"That's what you can call your chapter. Year One: Madness. Year Two: Madness the Sequel, because it was." In a local coffee shop, Vicki describes this time in her life to me. "I was overwhelmed, guilty and scared. I knew this wasn't going to go away or get better. I had to do something, but how could I take his car when it was his only connection to the world? How could I let him drive when it was so unsafe? He was easily lost already, and I was constantly watching the GPS and calling him." Vicki gifts him a cell phone with a tracker so she could find him. She reminds him to keep it with him at all times, and he is good about it. Lasiter, in fact, called quite frequently, forgetting he called her already.

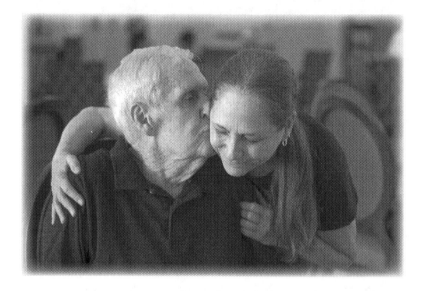

Faye and Vicki

We sip on our coffee, and she shakes her head saying, "I promised to have his back, and at the time I had to wonder what it even means." After a few beats of silence, "What was I supposed to do? I had no idea. I couldn't sleep. I couldn't think straight. I lived day to day and took care of whatever faced me. It was crazy land. I tried to not lose my patience and go nuts, but I'm here to tell you, it wasn't easy. I finally reached out to get some help, but this was not easy either. It wasn't easy for me at all. I failed him. That's how I felt."

> **"Remind yourself that the greatest technique for bringing peace into your life is to always choose being kind when you have a choice between being right or being kind."**
>
> **Wayne Dyer**

About the Lies...

Vicky visited various facilities not knowing what would be best for her father. The heartbreak over the situation was beyond anything she had dealt with in the past, and nothing seemed to be good enough for Lasiter. She was grateful when the executive director of one memory care facility was direct enough with recommendations and promises felt reasonable. Placement at a facility required some misleading stories and "lies" to guide Lasiter out of his house and into a place that he believed would be temporary. Vicki admits to becoming excellent at "lying" when it came time to take him to a place to live. "I'll own it. I'll deal with God. I had to do what was right for him, but it sure didn't feel right," she tells me. We both take a deep breath before she confides, "It didn't solve any problems either. It was better but still bad. I had to realize the kindest thing to do with dementia is to be dishonest"

> **"Glorify who you are today, do not condemn who you were yesterday, and dream of who you can be tomorrow."**
>
> **Neal Donald Walsch**

The New Normal

Vicki remains a constant figure in her father's life by spending long days with him at the facility and being in constant contact by phone. "If you open the window, there I was. If you turned to open the door, I was there too. I was everywhere," she laughs. Even so, Lasiter called her frequently asking her how long he needed to be there, when was he going to go home, and what happened to his car. The calls turn darker as he told her of his worry about one particular resident who was going into his room and taking his things. His feelings of persecution were amplified, and she was left to wonder what was happening. He didn't want to leave his room for fear someone would enter it and take his things, he refused to eat and his weight loss frightened Vicki. Securing a lock on his door was helpful, but the problems continued leading to physical altercations. She once again was left to make serious decisions. Vicki regretted placement but also knew he could not go back home. She was not able to care for him on her own. Regrettably, Lasiter lost his balance one day and fell resulting in hospitalization.

Vicki used the time away from the first facility to seek out an alternative. She knew there had to be a better option for her father. "I had to accept he would never be the same. I understood that. But he deserved to be better cared for. I had to be able to walk away and know he would be taken care of the way I would. I had to have that." And so it was.

Lasiter's body healed, but his dementia worsened following the injury and hospitalization. Vicki decided to take a chance with a memory care facility; so new Lasiter was one of the first residents. I photographed the arrival of the first four new residents, and this was when I met Vicki and Lasiter. Something simple, but momentous happened the first week to change the course for Vicki and Lasiter. Becca's smile, kind, and direct words lifted a weight and shifted Vicki's perspective. Becca was the facility's social worker. Vicki shared, "Becca asked me one day, 'why don't you let us do our jobs? We are here to take care of him. Your job is to love him.' I can't tell you how those few simple words moved me. It hasn't been easy, but I've released some of the control." Vicki proudly tells me she resisted visiting for a few weeks to let him adjust. She visits often but doesn't stay as long as she once did. She made friends with other families and no longer feels quite so alone on her journey. Vicki relinquishes some control to the staff that she has grown to trust and feels good knowing simply loving her father is often the best way to honor and protect him. Lasiter, now 94, enjoys his cup of morning coffee, the company of a dog named Brodie, and a daughter who always has his back.

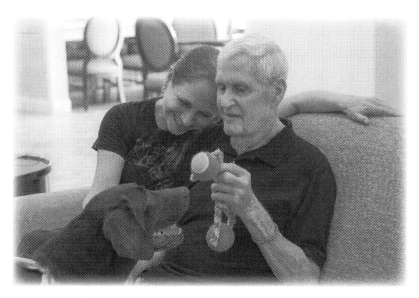

Faye, Vicki and Brodie

Six months have passed since I first met Vicki and Lasiter. Christmas lights, music, Santa Claus and plenty of good food surround us all. There is excitement in the air as families, residents, and staff enjoy the facility holiday party. I feel blessed to be there capturing love-filled moments with my camera. I notice Vicki and Lasiter sharing a conspiratory smile and shed a few happy tears as I catch a quick photo of their beautiful love. I am wrapped in Vicky's hug of gratitude knowing we have shared a very special time of her life neither of us will forget.

AFTERWORD

Vicki and Lasiter

Lasiter was one of the first residents when Poet's Walk Memory Care opened in Round Rock, Texas. Amber T., their Executive Director at the time was astute enough to value images and stories. She knew the importance of capturing a resident's first moments and first day at the facility as a way of welcoming them to their new home.

The images and stories can be healing for families. During our three hour session, I witnessed the anxiety and fear, the guilt, and the question of "did we make the right decision." Facility staff was warm and welcoming, and as the time passed the tension in their faces eased, and their smiles became genuine.

Vicky worried about every detail. There was no doubt she had experienced trauma as she cared for her 93-year-old father. She told me how she promised to "always have his back" but didn't know how to do this anymore.

We met for coffee a few weeks later to get to know one another. We talked for hours, and I loved her down to earth, straightforward, blunt approach. We went deep even questioning the presence of God. We asked one another the big questions and found our truths hidden away from a long time ago. As the disease progressed, her father's condition declined.

Months later and after considerable procrastination, I started my Facebook Live program, Carmen Talks Love, dedicated to telling the stories behind the images. It was a bold move for me because I was afraid to go live on social media. I committed to a date (Feb 7, 2017) and time to go live. I chose Vicky and Lasiter's story for my debut program, so I said a prayer, wrote an outline for the talk and sent messages to the facility staff and Vicky to let them know.

The Executive Director, Amber called to tell me how Lasiter had passed about the same time she received my message on February 6, 2017. I felt so bad about procrastinating. Why did I wait so long? I called Vicky to offer my condolences and asked her how she felt about a Facebook Live honoring her father. She wanted me to go forward and believed it was supposed to be this way. "I don't know much about this Facebook stuff, but it sounds like it would be a fine way to honor my Daddy." We all needed healing, and the timing couldn't have been better.

WILLIAM (BILL) BRITTON

I See The Joy

**We must let go of the life we planned, so as to accept
the one that is waiting for us.**

Joseph Campbell

Bill rode high on his accomplishments in sports and academics. He
held the esteemed position of quarterback for his El Paso high school
football team. The crowds roared them on as Bill, like many young
men, took on tackle after tackle to earn a win for their team. How
could he have known the actual price of those wins? The glimmer in
Bill's eyes is unmistakable as he describes his high school football days.
As if revealing for the first time, he looks around the table at his family
and me and says, "I was a quarterback, and loved playing the game."
He smiles broadly, "It was fun." He pauses as if just remembering, "I
got hit a lot, though and we didn't have much protection." He rubs the
side of his head before saying, "We didn't know anything like this could
happen. Nobody knew back then." The pride in his football memories
pale in comparison to the hardships clouding their lives today. They
didn't anticipate how the repetitive hits to his head in high school would
impact his still uncertain future.

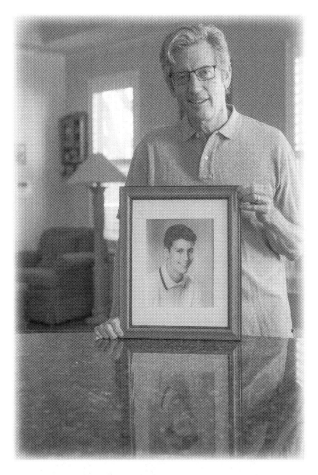

William

**Most of us have far more courage than we ever dreamed
we possessed**

Dale Carnegie

Bill developed a keen sense of what his wife Maureen calls business intuition
early on. "He knew what to do and when to do it. He became president of a
bank at age 28," she recalls. "He was so confident in his judgment and made
some risky decisions which paid off." Bill smiles and nods in agreement.
"He started working at age 14 and just kept climbing the ladder. We met in
college, didn't we Bill?" she asks. Although some of Bill's details are a little

off, giggles fill the room as they share their love story filled with conflict and resolution worthy of any romantic comedy film. Maureen pauses before stating, "He was highly respected, and when it happened, we were stunned." She takes a full inhale before revealing, "We were robbed. This is the honest truth. He was blindsided and railroaded by people he worked with and trusted. Living with the disease was all so much worse because he didn't need to lose his career so early on. He wasn't so bad off, and it was unfair losing his job and career. Our lives changed forever," tears fill her eyes. "I see couples our age living the life we should be living. We got robbed of it!"

Bill's high school football tackles are the suspected cause of his cognitive loss. At first glance, this would seem like the main culprit of Maureen's sense of loss. "I'm sorry" is a statement well known to the family. "Bill often tells me he is sorry, but it's not the same sorry I feel," Maureen pauses to look and smile at Bill. "I don't want him to blame himself. I blame people for how they treated him before we knew what was going on. I never blame him."

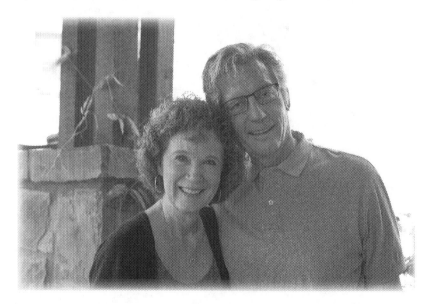

William and Maureen

At the age of 56, while many of us are considering retirement, welcoming grandchildren, or pondering a career change, Bill and Maureen faced a life altering crisis. Shaking her head in disgust, "We were stunned when he was put on medical leave from his work 'to get checked out' after one day he mistakenly called a client twice for the same purpose and didn't remember." She noticed some minor memory problems but blamed his long stressful work hours. While seeking medical support and assessment, they were devastated to find his employer didn't plan on his return. Subsequently, doors to others jobs within his career were 'slammed shut,' and his high paying career went flat overnight. Maureen laments, "We found out in such an odd way. We thought he was on leave long enough to see what was going on with him. It was not fair, and we were robbed of so much." They were stunned as their future took a sudden and dramatic turn. Maureen and Bill were unprepared for this new journey.

Making matters even more formidable, Bill's work up and the diagnosis was not an easy one for his physicians. While mild memory problems were evident to Maureen and others, he tested within average on cognitive tests because of his high baseline IQ. They eventually learned how his symptoms were likely the result of injuries he sustained playing football in high school. Bill was diagnosed with Traumatic Brain Injury (TBI) about 15 years ago. Although he had memory loss and other symptoms of dementia, dementia was not diagnosed until nearly a decade after his symptoms ended his career.

The family faced many lifestyle changes through the years. After losing his job, he was ostracized from jobs in banking and was never able to gain employment in his career. He held a variety of part-time positions and volunteer positions, but eventually, they became too difficult for him. They dramatically downsized their home, and Maureen changed companies for more job security with less time away from home. Bill no longer drives and relies on Maureen and other family members. Managing the television remotes, power switches and home appliances often requires assistance. Big and small changes turned Bill and Maureen's world upside down.

> **All great artists draw from the same resource: the human heart which tells us that we are all more alike than unalike.**
>
> **Maya Angelou**

Remember the Laughter

"You have no idea what it's like." Bill describes, "I feel like I have fuzz in my head. Especially in the morning. Their six-year-old grandson breezes over to share his thoughts, "The fuzz blocks up the memory. There's a giant bad guy in his head that puts a blanket over his head," he pauses to take a quick breath before continuing, "But when we play, it helps take the blanket away." He picks up a plastic design that looks like a peace sign and proudly states, "See, we made this. They're Perla Beads, and they're fun."

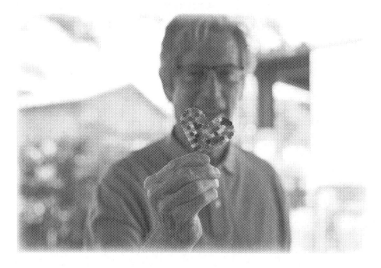

William

"Is this a peace sign, Bill?" I ask pointing holding up design. He proudly smiles, "It's steering wheel because it reminds me of when I could drive." He reaches through some other designs before handing over a heart shaped one, "I really like this one. It reminds me of laughter." Later in our visit, the family gathered for me to take their portraits, and I pick up the heart. "Bill," I say holding his heart design, "can I take your picture holding this?" A big smile washes across his face as he nods his head in affirmation. "Great! Thank you, Bill, I will look at it often so I too can be reminded of laughter."

Bill is a lover and a writer of poetry. "I think it was healing for him at first. He wrote some beautiful poems, and not all about dementia or his problems, but they tell his story. He has always been so smart, and we sometimes forgot just how creative he could be too," Maureen shares. It has become difficult for Bill to translate thoughts and feelings into words but he tells me he would like to try again. "The poems are so beautiful," Maureen laments. "I think about gathering them all up into a collection to be published. What do you think Bill?" Bill's face flashes with delight, "Yes I would." There is a pause to give him time to finish his thoughts, "I'm not sure why I don't write anymore, do you?" The air suddenly feels a tad thicker.

During our conversation, I ask Bill to describe himself. He is quick to tell me, "Resilient. I'm still here enjoying my kids," he waves to his son and family who sit with us. He and his grandsons openly discuss the variety of crafts and projects they enjoy. Bill also relishes in his daily walk with their dog Alfie and describes his favorite daily activity, "We walk to the park, and I throw the ball over and over again. It's so funny because Alfie enjoys it just the same every time." Bill continues to find his way to and from the park daily.

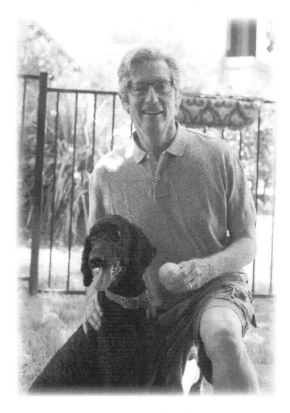

William and Alfie

There is a pause before one of his grandsons playfully squeals at one another from another room. Bill's son, Ryan, and daughter-in-law Nicki add, "Dementia has had a powerful effect on his emotions. It's harder for him to filter emotions. He sometimes gets frustrated with the kids, but amazingly, as his condition worsens, this has improved." They continue, "Little things get him so excited. It's as if each time is the first time, and things don't lose their appeal for him. He loves going to Costco and looking around. He is so excited to do crafts with the kids." Bill and his family gesture in agreement. Ryan adds, "He was always a joyful man, but he must've filtered out the happiness and joy. It was always there, but it stayed hidden away. He isn't able to suppress it anymore. I guess there is one good thing about the disease."

While the younger children roam in and out of the conversation, their 13-year-old granddaughter Veronica has been reluctant to join us. Unlike her younger siblings, she is old enough to remember Bill before dementia worsened. "It's just hard to think about this." She speaks through heart-wrenching sobs. After a bit, her mother Nicki adds, "She worries he won't remember her and the times they've had," Veronica sobs harder. "We all do, but it's hard for her to talk about it." My heart breaks a little as I try to filter my sadness.

The topic naturally flows to how they've learned to cope. His son Ryan asserts, "My sister and I make sure we know how things are, and we are both involved. She is further away, so she can't always be here, but we are all in contact." Maureen concurs. "I don't know what I would do without them. I sometimes worry about the burden on them, but they're the ones I turn to," she confides. "The grandchildren all know because we believe it is important they understand as best they can at their ages." Ryan and Nicki recall telling the children about their grandfather's condition, "Kids are pretty resilient and it wouldn't be right to pretend things are normal when they're not. They just need reminding once in awhile." While children are naturally resilient, it also seems to be a family trait.

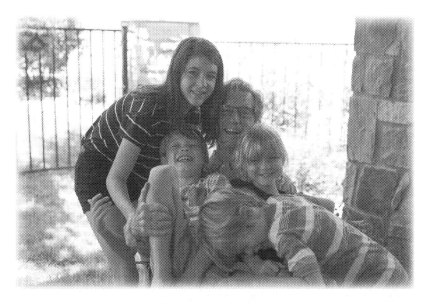

William and 4 of his 7 grandchildren

As our visit comes to a close, one of his grandsons runs up to me and excitedly says, "Oh yeah, this is important," he jumps in place a little, "He remembers us today, but he might not tomorrow. Did you know?" The air begins to condense a tiny bit more as the children go about playing. Bill smiles and Maureen hugs me goodbye. "I hope our story can help someone else," she whispers in my ear.

> **"Life is a series of natural and spontaneous changes. Don't resist them- that only creates sorrow. Let reality be reality. Let things flow naturally forward in whatever way they like,"**
>
> **Lao Tzu, a 6th century Chinese philosopher**

As I hug Maureen, I wonder if Tzu knew of the long, dry and winding path of dementia. Then I see Bill's big smile and consider perhaps Bill's pure joy in every new day, and his grandsons' acceptance of their reality is not a bad place to be today.

AFTERWORD

$\mathcal{B}$ill and Maureen

After working with Bill and Maureen at Seton Brain and Spine Institute Neurology Clinic, I told them I would be leaving the practice and why. Maureen cried because it takes time to know a medical provider and for them to know your story. I was grateful for the management of Seton to give me some scheduling flexibility so I could give a little more time when it was needed, and no one can blame Maureen for not wanting to start over.

She and Bill were interested in contributing to *Just See Me*. We made a date, and I met them at their home with their son, daughter-in-law and grandchildren. Her daughter and family who live in Chicago wanted to be there also, but were unable.

Bill's history of dementia is different than others with Alzheimer's Disease because of his history of head injuries when playing high school football. His symptoms began at a younger age, and Maureen was understandably struggling with the mountain of life changes and losses.

What I enjoyed most about my visit was hearing how Bill had always been kind but reserved his smile, laughter, and joy. His son told me how dementia seemed to lift the curtain and although his mother, Maureen has more burden, his father is happy, enjoying the simple things in life. They made me look at my life and responses to life's challenges a lot closer. I will be forever grateful.

Sadly, Bill died of complications of Alzheimer's Disease on November 17, 2017. Friends and family filled the pews. The stories they most loved telling were the ones demonstrating Bill's sense of humor and his love of play. Fear, heartbreak and questions over how this could happen weighed heavy as we celebrated a life well lived but cut short by dementia.

JACK L. THOMPSON

I'm Dying to be Forgiven

Forgiveness is the final form of love.

Reinhold Niebuhr

Bea walked by the activity room of the nursing home where she worked as a nurse and director of staff development. She glanced at the table in the corner and smiled as she saw her father, Jack L. Thompson play dominoes with three other residents. He is unable to speak more than a few words because of Parkinson's disease but is delighted. The father of seven grown children, he smiles to his daughter and waves as she walks by the room. He sees his daughter Bea most of every day, and his other children and grandchildren often. He still remembers them, though his memory is failing. She still feels his love even without his words."

Bea awakens after a restless night of sleep. She would not be able to go to work today and perhaps not any other day. "Daddy got sick, and then he died. This is the truth, and the rest is simply our stories," she groans in an unsuccessful attempt to soothe herself. Her imagination roams seeing his frail body loaded into the ambulance while his eyes ask her, "Why?"

No. Not today. The grief and the guilt bear down on her soul relentlessly. She could not go back.

Just a few months earlier, Bea awoke at 4 a.m. to bring her father coffee before returning home to prepare for her day. She again greeted him a few hours later to help him eat breakfast before assuming her role as LVN and director of staff development at New Hope Manor Nursing and Rehab Center in Cedar Park, TX. Bea loved seeing her father and observing his care and progress daily.

Bea's experience was much different before his arrival to New Hope Manor Nursing and Rehab Center and as his condition worsened, anger, resentment, powerlessness, and guilt fogged her mind. I like this better: The situations were beyond her control, but yet her heart broke. All she wanted was the best for her father's care.

"Life changes in the instant. The ordinary instant."

Joan Didion

Jack L. Thompson was in his eighties when a car accident unveiled the sad truth. Jack was no longer able to care for himself. He experienced physical and mental symptoms of Parkinson's disease with dementia-related communication and memory problems. Her father had been at New Hope Manor about two years after moving from a different facility. Shortly after the car accident, he lived five months with Bea's older sister where his care grew a bit more than they could handle. In spite of their vigilance, Jack continued to weaken.

Jack was an independent, hard-working father who didn't want or anticipate the help of his family. He, therefore, had no legal papers or plan for his ongoing care documented. As far as Bea knew, none of the seven siblings were legally assigned his physical or financial care until her older sister Sam stepped up to make decisions. They each experienced apprehensions and were not sure how to best care for their father. Bea felt betrayed, angry, resentful, and powerless when the family began to disintegrate as a result of poor communication and connection. Bea did not agree with all of Sam's decisions, though she knew Sam's intentions came from a place of love. "Nobody knew what was happening. We weren't sure what to ask. I kept thinking 'what would Daddy want' but I couldn't ask him," Bea said.

"All my life, I lived in the glory of others because I didn't feel I mattered"

Bea

Jack was married to Earnestine for 60 years. They had seven children and numerous grand and great-grandchildren. Jack served in the Army and was a Korean War Veteran. He provided for his large family and worked hard in construction. Bea was the second of six daughters and to the outside world appeared powerful and confident.

Bea hid her negative emotions much like she hid the anguish over a diagnosis of stage 4 breast cancer. She won her battle with cancer, but only showed the world the warrior Bea. The vulnerable, scared and lonely Bea remained hidden away. When Bea was seven, the family endured a house fire which destroyed their home and began a life Bea describes as lacking real joy and self-esteem.

Bea describes these experiences in her book, *Rise Up-Take Charge. Overcome. Succeed.* "We had wood stoves to keep us warm in the house, and one kerosene stove for cooking. I remember Mama warming water for our baths on the stove, and how good the water felt on my skin. We later warmed ourselves by the stove," Bea says with tears in her eyes. The stoves were sources of comfort and were central to their lives. One night when her father finished cooking, the flames on the kerosene stove unexpectedly continued to grow. "Go get me dirt! Now!" he yelled to the children. Her sister sprinkled her dirt on the flames, with no change. Bea continues, "I was a naive seven year old and ready to do my part. I would save the day! I sprinkled my dirt on the fire only to watch the blaze grow and swallow our home." The family was unhurt, but Bea felt responsible and secretly carried her scars on the inside. The burden of guilt weighed heavy on her spirit, and the shame kept her from ever mentioning it to her parents or siblings until near the end of her father's life. This pattern of silence continued in the family and eventually led to a slow destruction of their relationships.

When it came time to talk about the details of caring for Jack, there was little communication. "Daddy was in a car accident, and it became apparent he could no longer live on his own. My parents did not live together, and my sister who lived closest took over." Bea pauses before confiding, "I knew caregiving wasn't easy. I was the expert, but felt like my opinions didn't matter. I wanted to be involved in making decisions, and when I wasn't, I felt powerless." she continues. "I made sure everyone else had what they wanted and I put myself at the end of the line," she confesses.

"You know what else? I thought I had it together having been through some relationship breakups, raising my young grandson, and then breast cancer. I was tough, but my father's illness and death threw me to my knees," she confides. "When my sister took over the care and decisions, I knew she was in pain over Daddy's illness. I thought I was most loving by acknowledging her pain and going along with what she wanted." After a short pause, she continues, "I didn't realize how much I enjoyed being a more active part of his life until he came to live at New Hope Manor, and I saw him every day. He thrived, too. We were all involved in his care, and I gave weekly reports to everyone in hopes of improving all of our communication," she says.

Bea's eyes move toward the window as she sighs and confides, "It felt like a punch to me right here," she says pointing to her abdomen. "My greatest fear came true. My father was moved back to the first nursing home. I never even saw it coming, and I was destroyed." Bea silently cries and utters a muffled "I can still see it in mind. I can still feel it." What seemed like a betrayal and personal tragedy for Bea became the bridge leading toward a healthy, full life.

Sadly, Jack didn't make it to his new nursing home because he became seriously ill and the ambulance re-routed to the hospital. He almost died, but slowly recovered enough to leave the hospital and go to a nursing home. "When he was in the hospital, I had the chance to read the chapter of my book about the fire. I was so nervous because I had never said a word about my guilt," she recalls. "He couldn't talk, but he kept shaking his head as if to tell me it wasn't my fault," Bea holds her book in her hands. "It was as if 50 years of guilt lifted out of my heart in that instant," she snaps her fingers. "I knew I could focus on helping our family heal. I think on some level, Daddy understood this." There was a fire, and it burned down their house. The truth was undeniable. The blame Bea shouldered was her story, and the story was now over.

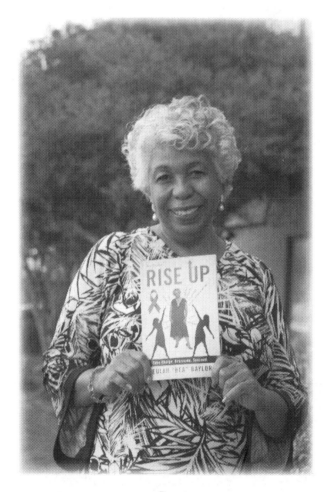

Bea

Jack died of a subsequent infection shortly after this hospital stay. "So many of us were there; all of his children, grandchildren, and great grandchildren were present. The crowd parted as my mother was rolled in next to him. It was like something out of a movie," she recalls. Jack was not awake and struggled with each breath. Bea gently guided her mother, "Mom, he knows you are here. Talk to him." Her mother leaned in and whispered in his ear, "Jack, you can go now. We are all here, and we will be okay." He took his last few breaths before passing.

"I decided it was the time I felt loved and appreciated, starting with me loving myself for a change." Bea, *Rise Up*

Bea spent months emotionally immobilized following her father's passing. Never able to return to New Hope Manor where memories of the last few days with her father lived, she was eventually able to take on some temporary staffing positions at other facilities. She invested time in finishing her book, taking care of herself, and attended self-empowerment workshops. "I woke up one day, looked into the mirror, and said, 'Ms. Bea, you matter. You are important too.' I meant it too," she says smiling.

> **"There is no love without forgiveness, and there is no forgiveness without love."**
> **Bryant H. McGill**

"I needed to forgive myself before I could think of reaching out to my sisters and brother. Our family needed healing. It had been long enough, and forgiveness was my goal. Daddy would want it for us too." The old patterns of silence no longer worked. "We create stories out of our lives, but these stories need to be broken down to the basics," Bea advises. "Daddy got sick, and then he died. The rest of it is my story or my sisters' or brother's stories. We all have a right to our story, but the only truth is the basic. He became sick and died. Realizing this helped me to love them deeper and heal from the pain, shame, guilt, and all those negative emotions."

Bea reached out to her family. They talked, cried, laughed, hugged, and eventually restored their family to the one Jack and Earnestine envisioned 60 years before.

AFTERWORD

$\mathcal{B}$ea and Jack

Bea and I are kindred spirits. We met through business acquaintances and share a hearty laugh and long career in nursing. I am grateful for Tonya Hofmann for suggesting I meet Bea even before I made the first pen stroke of this book. We became friends and our coffee hour (almost always 2-3 hours!) was a highlight for me. We shared business and personal triumphs and challenges. Over a year later I finished nearly all the interviews before Bea shyly told me her father had Parkinson's related dementia, and she had a story too. Yes, of course, there was room for her story!

When we sat down to talk about her father Jack and his illness and death, my level of respect for Bea rose even higher. The manner in which she handled the challenges with her siblings, the balance between being daughter and nurse and eventual transcendence and forgiveness is more than many of us will experience in our lifetime. This bright light is how she earned her title of *Queen Bea*.

We are sisters in our struggles to grow personally, professionally and spiritually. If only Jack could see how how his life and death formed his little girl into a beautiful, strong, and confident woman.

BILLIE S.

A Legacy of Loyalty

"You are on Earth because you have a job to do. Never doubt that." Billie may not remember her mother's words, but they continue to live in her heart. She strolls about believing she is at work nodding to her coworkers. Always quick to offer a hand, lead a spontaneous seminar, and tend to the typical workday tasks, Billie is content as she continues to make positive impacts on others. She doesn't realize she has dementia and lives in a memory care facility.

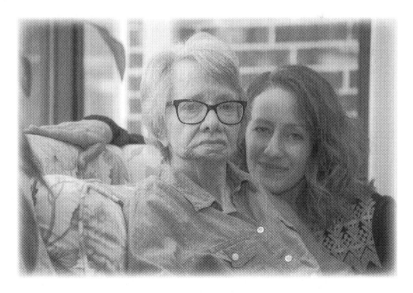

Billie and Laura

Staff members of Autumn Leaves memory care located in Northwest Austin offer whiteboards to each resident and help them to finish the statement: "I am…" They carefully wrote one or two-word descriptors such as "Happy" and "Sassy" and "A veteran." "Miss Billie, what do you want yours to say?" the young aide asked with her marker poised. Billie's face lit up with a sly smile as she proudly reported, "I am," she pauses and beams, "making change and not just at the register." A heartbeat of silence preceded an outburst of giggles and comments such as "that is just so Billie." Her wit and drive for social justice continue to flow even though she has dementia. Laura, her daughter, grins, "She likes being here because she believes she helps people. It hasn't made my decisions any easier though."

After being diagnosed at age four with cancer of the jaw, the medical treatments of 1940s radiated the right side of her face unaware of the dangers of high radiation. She lived with permanent scarring, deformity, and damage. Billie underwent 43 surgeries on her face only to discover breast cancer in her 50s. She recovered from each physical obstacle with her bright, quick-witted spirit intact. Every noble endeavor was a significant challenge and success until dementia began to chip away at her mind and spirit.

Billie earned a master's degree and taught college level English before earning a second master's degree in social work and becoming a social worker with hospice. With a passion for social change, she proudly worked with Martin Luther King and other activists. She eventually became Director of Social Work at her organization and won Social Worker of the Year in El Paso. Her heart was full while helping others in both big and small ways. She excelled as a realtor but didn't care for the work. "I believe she didn't like it because her clients sat to her right in the car, and she tired of feeling so self-conscious of her facial deformity," Laura, her daughter recalls. "Her success was proof the facial deformity was no competition for an outgoing, witty personality and smarts." A precocious professional working mother, Billie divorced Laura's father in the 1970s when divorce was not so common. She eventually remarried Lynn, a loving man who supported her activism and her dreams. "He loved us all so much and was so devoted to Mom," Laura recalls. "He was in awe of her as the incredibly well-rounded woman and loving mother. Her intelligence was something he noticed."

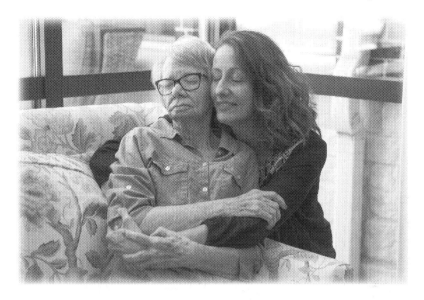

Billie and Laura

"Loyalty and devotion lead to bravery. Bravery leads to the spirit of self-sacrifice. The spirit of self-sacrifice creates trust in the power of love."

Morihei Ueshiba

Billie had her children's interests at heart and taught them the importance of family loyalty. Even as young children, she treated their opinions with respect. Airing opinions became teaching and bonding times for them. Above all, she taught them to always take care of one another. "We always have each others' back. Always," Laura shares, "It's a part of me as a wife, mother, and daughter. I care for a 16 year old and a 78 year old, and I worry about them all the time!" she laughs.

About ten years ago, Laura and her brother David noticed some changes in their mother. Her reasoning skills weren't as sharp as they had been and she became more forgetful each visit. Lynn didn't share his step children's concerns. "The decline was very slow. I don't think he saw it as we did and he certainly couldn't accept it," Laura says of her late step father. "Even when it was evident Mom was declining, he insisted on taking care of her at home. He was such a devoted man to her and all of us, but it became too much and borderline unsafe." Laura and David continued to stay in daily contact, a lifelong behavior. Laura smiles and confesses, "We are all high strung. We got that from Mom. We also inherited her sense of loyalty. There is no doubt we are there 100% for one another."

Being deeply loved by someone gives you strength while loving someone deeply gives you courage.

LaoTzu

The Turning Point

"Hello," Laura answers the phone still mostly asleep but recognizing the caller ID. "The police are on their way, but we thought you should know," her mother's neighbor reports. "Your mother is over here and says the man, her husband, is an imposter and not her husband at all." Laura is fully awake, and halfway out the door before the call is over.

"We weren't sure he could still take care of her," Laura remembers. "He insisted, but it was hard for him. We were close by, but they did things like eating out six to seven times a day because she forgot she had just eaten and he didn't want to tell her no. We intervened when it was necessary, but at the same time respecting their relationship." Lynn was at Billie's side until he had a serious car accident due to a diabetic crisis. He was severely hurt, but Billie recovered quickly. During this time, Laura and David made an excruciatingly painful decision and found a facility able to care for both Billie and Lynn once he recovered. During the eight months before his death, he visited Billie all day, every day. Her tiny body continued to diminish, and Billie needed care. Laura was overcome with grief and worry over doing the right thing when there were no good options. Billie no longer wanted to eat, and her health began to suffer. Following Lynn's passing, determined to help their mother, Laura and David decided to find a more suitable environment for Billie. After moving to Autumn Leaves, a memory care facility, she slowly started gaining her appetite and strength before becoming an active resident.

"The good life is one inspired by love and guided by knowledge."

Bertrand Russell

"I wasn't sure what to do. I promised her I would never put her in a home. I wanted to honor her wishes and take care of her at home with constant caregivers. I work full time and have a 16-year-old daughter and husband at home. Mom would be alone with the caregivers or me and would be so bored. She enjoys the company at the facility, and I watch over her very carefully, but I'm always, and I mean always wondering if I've made the right decisions." She pauses to wipe away a few stray tears. "I made a promise I thought I could keep, but in the end, I could not. Mom taught us loyalty, and I go around and around if I am loyal to her. Am I letting her down? I don't know. The concerns never leave my mind and heart."

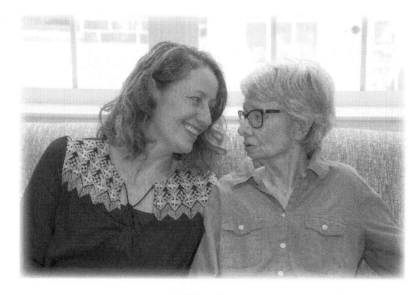

Billie and Laura

Shortly after her move to Autumn Leaves memory care, she gained weight and strength, and no longer needed hospice. It is uncommon for people with advanced dementia to improve while on hospice but Billie's spirit prevailed. She is interested in conversations with other residents, but she is most fond of interacting with the staff who she believes is her work colleagues. Billie can be found leading a spontaneous workshop for residents as they watch TV while other days she is busy folding clothes. She has been known to offer raises to the staff in appreciation of their service.

The Face of Loyalty

Laura and her brother David visit their mother every day. They've developed relationships with the staff who are quick to text or call if there is anything out of the ordinary. "My mother taught me about loyalty and about always, always having each others' backs. The hard part I thought was it meant I would keep my promise to take care of her at home, but now maybe it means I visit her often and make sure she is taken care of as she deserves. There are staffing fluctuations, and I believe people who care for our elderly are underpaid. The situation is not great anywhere, but it's just the way things are. They do a good job, but I worry all the time. I wonder if I have made the right decisions, all the time. It never leaves me."

"I know there will come a day when she won't recognize me," Laura tears up. "I'm going to love on her even though she won't know me. Maybe that'll scare her. I've seen that too. A heart attack or other sudden death would be a miracle at this point. We don't have a way to medicate for emotional and spiritual pain like we can physical pain. She would not want to live like this. She told me so many times, and yet this is all I can do for her." Families left to watch the physical and mental decline often suffer deep emotional pain as they watch and wait.

'Sometimes the heart sees what is invisible to the eye."

H. Jackson Brown, Jr.

Today is a good day. We met with Billie shortly after our chat. Billie is happy to see her Laura and eager to shake my hand as we enter. I address her as a colleague, and ask if I could take a few photographs of her. She laughs a little and asks, "What do I do?" I tell her, "You just be yourself, Billie. It'll be perfect." She is quick to say, "No problem. I'm an expert."

She beamed with joy at the prospect of helping me complete my project. She never tired even though we took pictures in a variety of places around the facility. She gave me some directions by suggesting where I might stand and where we might go next, and offer other residents the opportunity to join her. "Why are you doing this again?" she repeated.

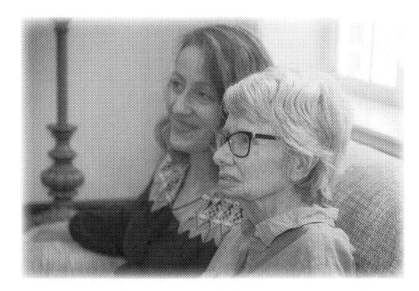

Billie and Laura

I couldn't help but notice Billie had no reluctance to smile or have the right side of her face toward the camera. She was no longer a camera shy beautiful lady with self-conscious worries about her facial deformity. Scars which once brought such angst seemed to become badges of honor and strength. Billie was once full of wisdom, and powerful language which created change. Her willingness to show her physical scars demonstrated strength beyond words. Once we finished, I gave her a big hug, and she said, "you work so hard. I'm going to put you in for a raise." This kindness and generosity are the reasons why Billie is so loved. She didn't complain about being tired or about the many photos I snapped but instead complimented me. Her second hug was a bit tighter, and I was the one wiping away tears.

AFTERWORD

Billie and Laura

Meeting Laura and Billie in the clinic at Seton Brain and Spine Institute was a blessing. They were sad to hear of my leaving the practice and yet reluctantly eager to contribute Billie's story. Laura wasn't sure if their story could help someone else, but was willing to take a chance.

I remember the complicated history and the loving way Laura, her daughter, weighed heavy with guilt over every decision, struggled to do what was most respectful yet safe for her mother. The fatigue and stress showed as did her loving, warm heart.

After hearing Laura's stories of growing up with Billie who instilled a strong sense of family loyalty, I saw Billie in a new way. She was always clearly intelligent, welcoming but astute, and blunt but kind. I also recognized the exceptional mother she continues to be.

In the summer of 2017, I went to see Laura and Billie who was at Hospice Austin's Christopher House. Billie laid pale, weak and frail in a bed of white linens. She hadn't been able to eat in days. Laura and I chatted for a while as she slept. When it was time for me to go, I went over to hold Billie's hand, and she awoke. Laura let her know I had come to visit.

"Well, hi Carmen. How are you? Is there anything I can get for you?" she said before closing her eyes again. "No Billie. You've given me quite enough." Billie rallied, began eating again and though still frail, she was able to leave the hospice facility. She now resides in assisted living at Poet's Walk Cedar Park.

JOHN B

Running for My Life

"Do not dwell in the past, do not dream of the future, concentrate the mind on the present moment."

Buddha

John and Becky lived an enviable life. Happily married for 41 years, they built a life with three children, successful careers, and exotic travel. Becky is an attorney with her own firm, while John was an economics professor. Their plans for retirement included a busy social and travel calendar until dementia changed things.

Every morning, John prepares his cereal and coffee while Becky watches. "The milk is in the refrigerator John," she prompts when he appears troubled. Each time he needs more cues, Becky's heart skips a beat. He slowly opens the door and retrieves the milk, "Thank you. I sometimes forget things." She nods and sips her coffee, "I know honey. It's okay." He finishes his breakfast, rinses the dishes, and puts them in the dishwasher.

"What is next John?" she asks. He looks at their two cats Clancy and Cleo and is reminded of his daily routine, "I need to feed them," he points. He looks around the room not sure where they keep the cat food, and Becky resists the urge to provide guidance. "It's in here," he proudly proclaims. She feels a profound sense of gratitude in this moment.

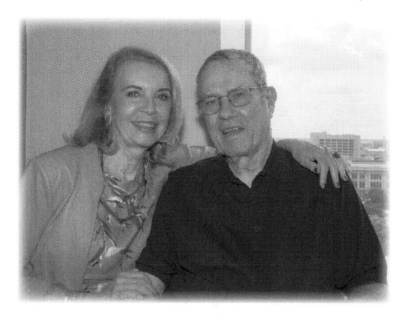

John and Becky

"Learn from yesterday, live for today, hope for tomorrow. The important thing is not to stop questioning."

Albert Einstein

John and Becky love to travel with their family. Their son Matt lives nearby, and in spite of John's memory problems, they have been able to travel to see their daughter Jennifer and another son Will.

"We have visited 30 countries including five trips to Africa since his diagnosis ten years ago," Becky shares. She asks John if he can name the countries they've visited. After a short struggle, he says, "I get a little forgetful sometimes." She nods and pats his hand. "He loves to travel and does well with it. I know most people slowly get worse with dementia, but John has been about the same for ten years. We've noticed a decline the past year though."

Becky proudly describes John as incredibly smart with an understated dry wit. "He worked on cars, built things, read religiously, and loved crossword puzzles. Fifteen years ago when he was 65 years old, we noticed he couldn't spell simple words, and I knew something was seriously wrong. He didn't understand concepts like recycling and couldn't work the remotes anymore." John's problems began about the same time he retired from teaching, and some physicians first believed depression was to blame. "With such a high IQ, he scored well on the tests, but we all knew this was well below his normal." This frustrating time lasted about four years before specialists diagnosed him with Alzheimer's disease, a type of dementia.

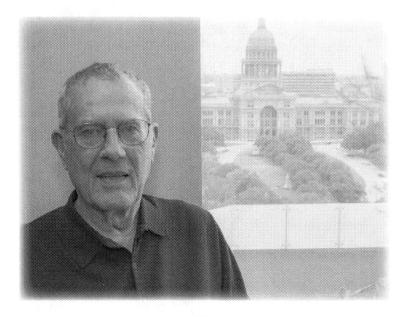

John

"Have patience with all things, but, first of all with yourself."

Saint Francis DeSales

While John is understated, Becky is high energy in her professional and personal life. She views problems as challenges to overcome and relies on the support of her friends, family, hired caregivers, and colleagues. "I know I am lucky to have the network I do. When I have questions or John needs to see a specialist, I make a phone call. Many people don't have this," she confides.

Becky is clear about her caregiving role, "You've got to have some help and time for yourself. Sandra, John's daytime caregiver, is a lifesaver. She stays with John every day, so I can work and even stays late, if needed. They have a routine with meals and errands, and she often brings him downtown to my office. Everyone here," she waves to her multi-office suite law firm, "know about John and are very good to him." Becky looks to Sandra, "I am fortunate to know he is well cared for even when I'm not there." John and Becky spend two to three evenings a week attending galas, parties, eating out, and enjoying live music. She notes, "John enjoys going out. As long as he can see me, he does amazingly well in a crowd, and he loves to eat out," Sandra adds.

Every Day is a New Day

When John's symptoms of Alzheimer's disease started about fifteen years ago, Becky was scared. "There I was, confident and fearless until I faced dementia. I constantly wondered if I was doing the right thing. Every day is a new day with dementia and what worked yesterday may not work today. People gave me tips, but I had to figure it out for myself. The first three things may not work, but I figured it out."

Becky continues, "I can anticipate our day based on the morning. There are three general categories: Happy and cooperative, angry and oppositional or confused with a mix of angry and happy." Becky confides, "It's sad, but as his memory worsens his mood improves because he can't remember why he was angry."

Take Care of Yourself

Becky learned to be a better wife and caregiver by taking care of herself. "I had to make sure I had time for myself not being a caregiver." Becky works more than full time in her law practice and is active in over twenty non-profit organizations. "I'm very high energy with minimal downtime. This is my diversion from caregiving and helps me cope. Every caregiver needs to find how they cope best and do it."

Becky was recently named Outstanding Caregiver of the Year by Alzheimer's Texas where she delivered a moving speech about her vulnerabilities as a caregiver. "The week before the Alzheimer's Texas Hidden Heroes luncheon, John was so agitated and confused, and I was worried," she exclaims. "We had a doctor's appointment right after the luncheon. Once we stopped one of his longtime medicines, he did better." She repeats with emphasis, "Every day is a new day."

Giving Choices and Making Decisions

Even with Becky's ample resources, it is still complicated caring for a loved one with dementia. "I approach problems with logic. In the beginning, I tried to reason with him, and this did not work. I had to train myself to agree and redirect, but it took time." While two of John and Becky's adult children live out of state, their son Matt lives closer. "I call our son Matt the *Dad Whisperer* because he is good at de-escalating and figuring out what to suggest to make everybody happy. We give John choices and encourage him to make decisions. When his decision isn't good, such as when he insists on wearing his tux shoes to the running track, we jump in," Becky says as she and Sandra share an appreciative glance.

> **"We keep busy. Keeping your mind and your body active is important. This is John's Golden Key."**
>
> **Becky**

John has been a runner most of his life having participated in a variety of full marathons including New York, Boston, and many others. "It is important to stay active. I think this is why he has done well. He pushes himself with his trainer Randeen. They run a mile on Town Lake in Austin two to three days a week.

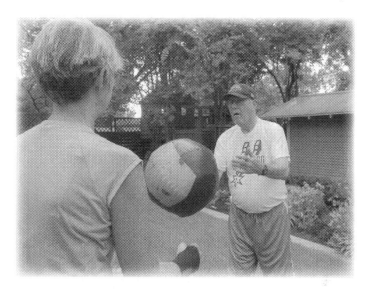

John and his trainer Randeen

This routine is good for him. On the days he doesn't run, they do flexibility and weight training at home. He is still very good at following directions," she proudly admits. "The worst thing people can do is stop being active and sit around. The brain and the body have to stay active. The doctors are impressed with how great John is doing, and I know strenuous exercise is John's Golden Key."

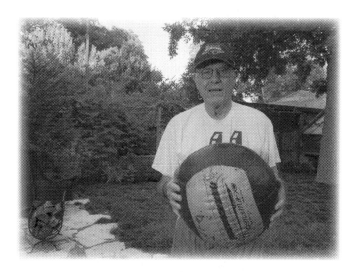

John

"Worry never robs tomorrow of its sorrow; it only saps today of its joy."

Leo Buscaglia

"I don't worry much because when there is a problem, I just solve it," Becky declares. "I had to think about my mortality when I had breast cancer. For the first time, I had to consider how to care for John if I couldn't anymore. I'm cancer free, and we caught it early, but it made me think about my life. I took action, and we prepared a legal plan," Becky confides.

"My big concern is the risk of falls. While on vacation in Argentina, he fell on a familiar path because he thought the shadows on the walking path were holes. He wasn't hurt, but he fell," she clarifies. "I know when someone falls, things get much worse, and I can't imagine this happening." Now she is more vigilant when they walk, and he and his trainer do balance exercises. She pauses to glance my way, "Sometimes he shuffles a little. This scares me so much."

"Grief is in two parts. The first is the loss. The second is the remaking of life."

Anne Roiphe

In spite of her many resources, Becky admits to feeling lonely. "I am lonely for the life I expected. We planned National Geographic travel for our retirement." Becky paused and gathered her thoughts, "Plans changed, and I was sad when he couldn't help me redraft our future."

While their future is uncertain, one fact remains for Becky, "I'll keep working, and having fun because this is how I cope." She reaches over and places her hands over John's, "We do fine don't we?" He smiles and after a pause, "Yes I believe so. I just forget things sometimes."

AFTERWORD

John and Becky

Becky gave a moving speech at an Alzheimer's Texas luncheon honoring caregivers. She is a pillar of strength and I was moved when she acknowledged her fears and vulnerabilities. I couldn't help but think how many of us would feel some release of pressure trying to be the perfect caregiver when we saw this beautiful, confident woman confess her feelings of inadequacy as a caregiver.

She worries about their future and grieves their plans. She reminds us Alzheimer's Disease and other dementias can happen to anyone and indeed it does. Becky's coping response to a scary disease was to jump into action, learn to take care of her husband while honoring her need for self-preservation.

There is so much I love about Becky's story, but my favorite is her reminder that we don't have all the answers but by living the experience we find them for ourselves. I'm a 'take action' lady also, and respect Becky for her unique power and vulnerability.

JUDY

How Do Other People Do This?

"We are a very private family. You honor my mother by sharing her story for our family. Some people who live right near us didn't even know about the Alzheimer's."

Roxanne, Judy's daughter

Judy's history in the small community of Noack, Texas with its population of 100 is narrow, but deep. She grew up among the rolling hills of ranches and farms before marrying and raising her six children. Judy lovingly managed a busy household and helped her husband Elton build a thriving business.

Judy's grown children live nearby and most work in the family business. Her daughter Roxanne tends to her mother's care and manages the household. "We all worked hard on the farm and in the fields growing up," Roxanne begins. "Momma was born into a hard-working family and started young. She could pick up a big sack of cotton and swing it around over her shoulders like it was nothing. We worked the farm early in the morning and then made lunch for the boys," she pauses and smiles. "After we made lunch and the guys went back out, we watched The Young and the Restless, As the World Turns, and Guiding Light before starting the other chores. When I was growing up, one of my favorite memories was watching the Soaps with Momma."

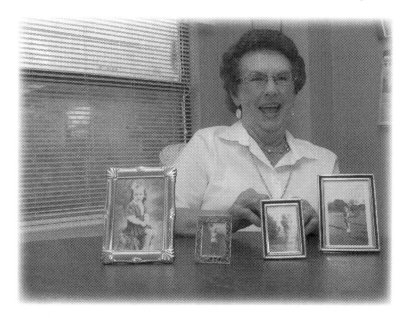

Judy

How Do Other People Do It?

Roxanne tends to her mother's care and manages the household daily.

Roxanne and Judy have a nightly routine since her mother's Alzheimer's disease has worsened. "Have you brushed your teeth, Mother?" Judy asks knowing reminders work better than requests. They complete their rituals, and Roxanne says, "Tomorrow is Sunday Momma." Roxanne smiles as she waits for her mother's typical bright response, "Sunday? Church day!" Roxanne nods as she savors her mother's joy and simultaneously dreads the day Judy will not remember how much she loves Sundays.

Once her parents are tucked in, Roxanne drives the short distance home trying to slow her racing mind. The daily tasks of caring for her children, her husband, the farm, and her parents sometimes take a toll. The responsibilities have grown as her mother's health has deteriorated. "I sometimes don't know how I'll do it. What do other people do?" she wonders out loud.

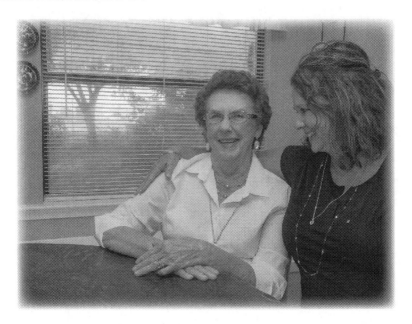

Judy and Roxanne

"It is important for all of us to appreciate where we come from and how that history has really shaped us in ways we might not understand."

Sonia Sotomayor

In a bright green field, Christ Lutheran Church stands tall on a foundation of family values. The tall steeple stands guard over the tiny community. Judy has been Superintendent of Sunday School for over 50 years. She still holds this title even though she is unable to fulfill the role anymore.

As we walk through the Sunday School area, Roxanne points out, "This is a picture of you Momma with your confirmation class when you were twelve. It was taken right here where we are tonight." Judy proudly looks at the large image pointing to her face and smiles, "This is me. That was a long time ago though."

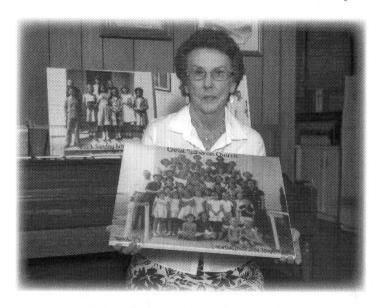

Judy with Photo of her Confirmation Class

We walk along the sacred grounds of the church as Roxanne shares some history, "Momma has been active in the church since she was born. Her great-grandfather donated the land 125 years ago so German immigrants could have a place to worship. Her family helped build it."

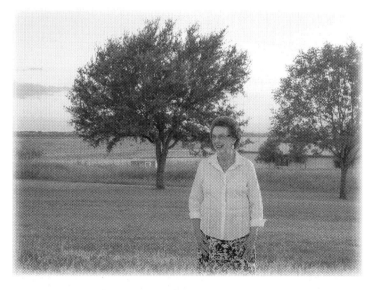

Judy on the grounds of Christ Lutheran Church

They pose by the newly acquired historical marker, "Momma can't tell you what day it is or remember what happened five minutes ago, but she can tell you details about church events from her childhood. I get to see my real Momma when I bring her here. You know?" Roxanna wipes away a tear.

> **"Emotional discomfort, when accepted, rises, crests and falls in a series of waves. Each wave washes a part of us away and deposits treasures we never imagined. Out goes naïveté, in comes wisdom; out goes anger, in comes discernment; out goes despair, in comes kindness. No one would call it easy, but the rhythm of emotional pain we learn to tolerate is natural, constructive and expansive... The pain leaves you healthier than it found you."**
>
> **Martha Beck**

"About eight years ago, I knew something was wrong when she started to do some strange things," Roxanne pauses to ask her mother, "This isn't easy to talk about is it Momma?" Judy who sits next to us, demurely smiles and nods, "Oh, it's okay I guess."

Roxanne continues, "It has been really hard for all of us including Momma, and we don't always see things the same. Daddy didn't notice for a long time, and it was hard to get an answer from the doctors."

Seven years ago, Judy saw her family physician after Roxanne noticed her mother was driving dangerously, had troubles with routine tasks, and placed unusual things in the refrigerator. At the time, the doctors reassured them the changes were normal for a 71-year-old woman.

"Momma was still babysitting the younger grandchildren, and I just didn't feel right about it, so I was here more and more. I didn't think she should drive anymore, but this was hard to talk about," Roxanne says. "She hurt her knee, so I started driving her around. She never asked about driving again, which was a good thing."

About four years ago, Roxanne recognized it had become unsafe for Judy to be alone during the day and assumed the caretaker role. Judy was eventually diagnosed and began treatment for Alzheimer's disease, a type of dementia, a year later.

Judy needs guidance and supervision for most things, and the family has rallied to help. Her daughter, Cheryl makes breakfast for her parents every morning and often throws in a load of laundry. Roxanne arrives shortly after, tends to her mother and maintains the family home throughout the day. "I take care of my parent's house, the shopping, laundry, and cooking, and then go home and do the same for my family," Roxanne confides. "Momma is usually agreeable, but she doesn't always understand, and there can be resistance."

Roxanne shares some frustrations of caregiving, "I've learned how to manage. I don't always expect the changes either. Unless people are here and see it, they can't understand how hard it is. Who could I even turn to for help?"

> **"Hope lies in having more faith in the power of God to heal us than in the power of anything to hurt or destroy us. In realizing as children of God we are bigger than our problems, we have the power at last to confront them."**
>
> **Marianne Williamson**

Like many caregivers of those with dementia, Roxanne has health problems. "I know the good Lord is with me all the time. I have faith, but I sometimes get so busy I forget to pray. I ask God for help all day as I work, but I don't take quiet time to myself to pray anymore," she confides. "Even though I'm on auto-pilot and overwhelmed, the good Lord is first, and I want to remember to pray and ask for what I need."

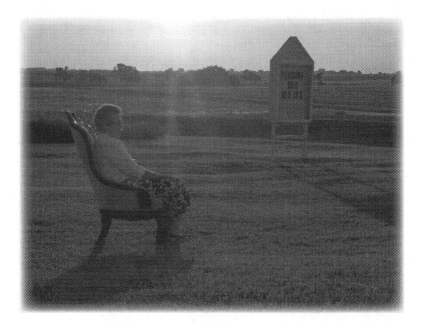

Judy on the grounds of Christ Lutheran Church

Roxanne is quick to describe the joy of caring for her family even when feeling physically and emotionally exhausted. "When I'm not here, I'm thinking about it. I love and honor my parents and can't even consider another way to do this," she confesses. "There are days I hurt so bad I can hardly get out of bed but so long as I can keep this up, I will."

> **"Consciously or not, we are all on a quest for answers, trying to learn the lessons of life. We grapple with fear and guilt. We search for meaning, love, and power. We try to understand fear, loss, and time. We seek to discover who we are and how we can become truly happy."**
>
> **Elisabeth Kubler-Ross**

Roxanne's son is a healthcare administrator of a long-term care facility.

Roxanne thinks about her future, "If I get Alzheimer's disease, I would love for them to care for me on a daily basis like I do Momma. Even with financial support, they would still have the physical and emotional pain knowing what is happening to me," she says. "Honestly, I just crave peace with no worries or expectations."

"You can love someone so much... But you can never love people as much as you can miss them."
John Green

Roxanne has a variety of health problems and significant physical pain, but the emotional distress of caregiving is the most challenging. "I know I have to come to terms with the reality of dementia. Sometimes she has a clear moment, and I feel hopeful how maybe she doesn't have Alzheimer's after all," she says. "Then disappointment and reality hit me. How can I miss her so much even though she is right next to me," she discreetly wipes away a tear while reaching for her mother's hand. Judy silently holds Roxanne's hand and clearly recognizes her daughter's sorrow.

Roxanne enjoys Judy's smiles and giggles as they look through old photos. "I remember her. What's her name?" Judy asks repetitively. She often remembers events and the love they shared but not the details.

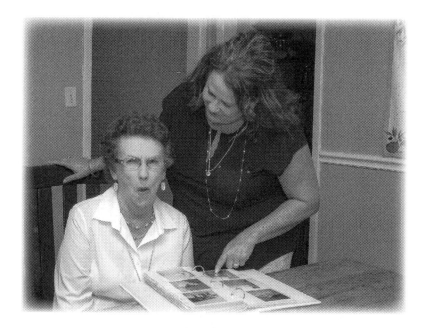

Judy and Roxanne

Later in the day, Judy is proud to show me around their beloved church as I snap pictures. We step back in time, and I catch glimpses of Judy and Roxanne and the miracle of love.

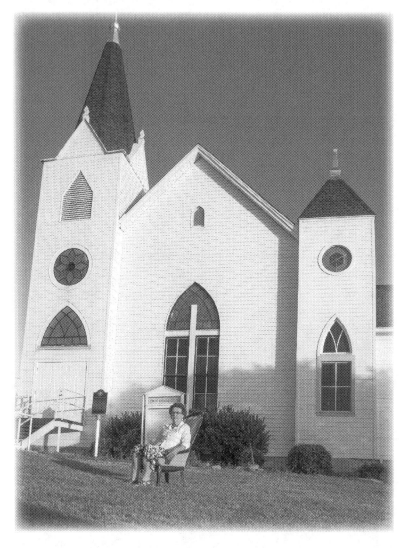

Judy on the grounds of Christ Lutheran Church

AFTERWORD

Roxanne and Judy

Roxanne and Judy's inclusion in this book was divine intervention. We met initially at the Seton Brain and Spine Institute Neurology Clinic in Austin, TX where I did my best to help Roxanne navigate around the challenges of caregiving. They had the added difficulty of living in the country on the family farm. Roxanne became the family spokesperson doing her best to explain to the others what was happening to her mother, the family matriarch while doing her best to care for her husband and children.

Months after I left the clinical practice, I ran into Roxanne and Judy having lunch at a local restaurant. None of us go out to lunch often, so it was quite the coincidence. Roxanne asked me about the book and let me know they would like to contribute if there was still room. I planned to cap it at the 10 stories I had already finished so I told her there was no more room. I could laugh at my naiveté now since I was nowhere near done and it took me a year to write the stories. She gave me her contact info, and we went our different ways. I planned to contact them if things changed, but time got the best of me, and her contact information was lost in the shuffle. I'm not proud of this, but it is the truth.

As the next year passed, I finished the interviews and photos, and it became evident how the stories were evolving to truly sacred stories of the families' legacies. This evolution meant it would take more time, and it was all worth it.

I was busy with editors, business coaches, website designers and others while building my photography business. My hours typically started at 8 am, and I closed the computer around 1or 2 am every day, and yet I rarely felt fatigued because storytelling and photography became my mission. Yes, it was 'Mission from God' as I explained in the Preface. However, the book completion day kept getting moved further and further into the future.

Over the summer as I wrapped up the last story, I received a text I didn't recognize. I inquired, and Roxanne admitted to accidentally texting me instead of her daughter's friend also named Carmen. She wrote: "I know last summer you said you were at the end and I wish you could've featured Mom in there, but you said you were finishing up. But that was last summer."

I saved her texts because they remind me how there are times when God gives you nudges and other times when you get a good swift kick in the pants. This was my kick. At first, I felt such shame, but it was quickly replaced with an intense knowing how Judy and Roxanne's story just had to be in the book.

When Judy showed me around her church with such clarity and brilliant joy, I found myself very grateful for auto-focus because my eyes were too teared up to otherwise focus my camera. The book wouldn't be the same without Roxanne's touching raw description of being thrust into the caregiving role and the toll it has taken on her. Learning about their story truly touched my life and heart in ways I could not have imagined. There are no coincidences. It was meant to be.

AFTERWORD

Just See Me-Sacred Stories from the Other Side of Dementia

I hope you enjoyed reading *"Just See Me-Sacred Stories from the Other Side of Dementia."* I see it as a variety of beautiful threads and textures all coming together and perfectly woven to become a beautiful cloth. It represents every story, every soul, all the support, every hurdle and also the final product which you hold in your hands.

We are all caregivers.

Some of us provide loving care by choice, while others wake up in an unfamiliar world and want to throw the pillow over our heads. Some of us care for our families, our businesses and hopefully ourselves, and yet we each approach the tasks differently. While providing loving care may seem inherently 'built- in' simply because we are all human beings, any caregiver will tell you there is a lot to learn. Check out some super resources out and a variety of information right here: At https://www.CarmenBuck.com.

Tough Caregiver Concerns

- What do you need to know to take care of someone else?
- Do you want to be a caregiver?

- How would you like to define your caregiving role?
- Is there such a thing as balance?
- I hear about the holistic approach-body, mind and spirit but don't really know much about it.
- What if I harbor resentment?
- What if the person needing care pushes me away?

I'm there to offer support, guidance and big reminders of the importance of self-care along the way. During my own experiences of being a caregiver (some by choice and others with my heels dug in very deep!) I found self-care to be the most challenging aspect. So, I'm here for you! Be sure and check it out.

One Simple Path

You can find your way as a caregiver by reaching out for help along the way. Let the stories of *"Just See Me"* be a guide.

Whether you are a caregiver or not, please consider the little things you can do for others. As you walk down the street, pass cars on the road, check out at the grocery story and so on, remember how every person you meet carries their own burden. Offer a smile, a hand, a compliment or other act of kindness. Be present for one another. There is no greater gift than the love woven into the following words: "I'm here. I'm listening."

You Are Not Alone

We learn from one another when we, as caregivers, open our doors and hearts and authentically admit to the difficulties and the joys. Our world, even if it isn't quite what we imagined, becomes larger and more delightful when we let the truth out.

Visit https://www.CarmenBuck.com for upcoming webinars, free newsletters, special Facebook groups, E-books and so much more for caregivers of any kind.

Printed in the United States
By Bookmasters